# A Garden
of Unearthly Delights

*Robin Mather*

# *A Garden of Unearthly Delights*

*Bioengineering
and the Future
of Food*

A DUTTON BOOK

DUTTON

*Published by the Penguin Group*

*Penguin Books USA Inc., 375 Hudson Street, New York, New York 10014, U. S. A.*
*Penguin Books Ltd, 27 Wrights Lane, London W8 5TZ, England*
*Penguin Books Australia Ltd, Ringwood, Victoria, Australia*
*Penguin Books Canada Ltd, 10 Alcorn Avenue,*
*Toronto, Ontario, Canada, M4V 3B2*
*Penguin Books (N.Z.) Ltd, 182–190 Wairau Road, Auckland 10, New Zealand*

*Penguin Books Ltd, Registered Offices:*
*Harmondsworth, Middlesex, England*

*First published by Dutton, an imprint of Dutton Signet,*
*a division of Penguin Books USA Inc.*
*Distributed in Canada by McClelland & Stewart Inc.*

*First Printing, June, 1995*
*1 3 5 7 9 10 8 6 4 2*

 REGISTERED TRADEMARK—MARCA REGISTRADA

LIBRARY OF CONGRESS CATALOGING-IN-PUBLICATION DATA

Mather, Robin.
A garden of unearthly delights : bioengineering and the future of food / Robin Mather.
p. cm.
"A Dutton book."
Includes index.
ISBN 0-525-93864-8 (acid-free)
1. Agricultural biotechnology. 2. Food—Biotechnology. 3. Food. 4. Nutrition. I. Title
S494.5.B563M38 1995
338.1'9—dc20 94-47367
CIP

*Printed in the United States of America*
*Set in Bauer Bodoni*

*Designed by Steven N. Stathakis*

*for my father,*
*Robert Bates Mather*
*(1918–1978)*

# *Acknowledgments*

The thought and counsel of many people helped shape my opinions as I researched this book. It is impossible to name them all for fear of leaving someone out. To them I owe profound gratitude, but I retain responsibility for all errors.

Thanks go to:

Lisa Ross of the Spieler Agency, Carole DeSanti of Dutton, and Rachel Klayman for believing that others share our concerns about the way food is produced.

Bill and Kitty Liebhardt for patience, a fine meal, and the generous sharing of the passions of two lions' hearts.

Robert Giles, Julia Heaberlin, Martin Fischhoff, David Good, Lynda Page, Dia Pearce, Diane Hofsess, Susan Whitall, Scott Martelle, Robert Ourlian, Reed Johnson, and Marla Dickerson, all of *The Detroit News*, for clearing the decks so I could write and/or for reading with an intent eye what I have written.

Sam and JJ Prestridge for pressing me to search out the eternal verities in french fries—so I could explain them to you. We'll talk.

Michael Knobler for his seeming belief that I walk on water. He has sometimes convinced even me that I can—once or twice.

Felder Rushing for things too numerous—and sometimes too scandalous—to mention.

Beverly Bundy and Ruth Larsen for always listening with open hearts and open minds.

Joseph Gray and Desmond Toups for an undismissible debt of boundless friendship, boundless faith, and boundless courage.

Sally and Timmy McCarthy for a kind of open-handed, open-hearted love that is simply astonishing.

My little brother Steve G. for playing the catalog game those many years ago. He is Mr. Archives and Records, a tireless rooter-on, the proud clipper of my columns, and the possessor of a smile as warm as the sun.

Mark and Michael and Wheaten, my sons-by-proxy.

And Judith Schneider, because there are not words enough in the hearts of man to thank you adequately.

# Contents

# *Introduction*

"Hey, honey," my silver-haired mother said from the easy chair in her living room. "I got this sample of cappuccino in the mail. Do you want some? Let me read you the ingredients."

She put on her reading glasses, and still she had to squint to read the list.

"Let's see: sugar, nondairy creamer (with partially hydrogenated soybean oil), maltodextrin (from corn), sodium caseinate (from milk), dipotassium phosphate, mono- and diglycerides, soy lecithin, instant coffee, cocoa (processed with alkali), sodium citrate, and artificial and natural flavor."

We looked at each other for a moment before bursting into laughter.

"Gee, Mom," I said. "That sounds just *yummy.*"

"Remember when coffee was made from roasted coffee

beans?" she asked. "And if you wanted milk and sugar in it, you added it yourself? Whatever happened to those days?"

David Tricoli exhales a puff of frustration as he surveys his failures, which far outnumber his successes.

One failure, on a bed of agar in its lidded petri dish, looks like a couple of tablespoons of premasticated lime Jell-O: frothy, bubbly, pale translucent green, sort of wiggly.

Another looks vaguely plantlike: it's deep green and spiky, like a bit of chewed grass.

Still another is a real disappointment: with no chlorophyll at all, it looks like the foam that dish detergent makes in hot water.

"They just don't have the plant structure we need," mutters David.

In his white lab coat, its tails flaring like the wings of angels, he strides away from his disappointments.

David, a plant geneticist for the Upjohn Company's agricultural division, is struggling to create something for your dinner table. He's working on a transgenic squash—a squash that has genetic material from several viruses added to the squash's DNA. That "vaccination" at a genetic level will help the squash plant resist diseases. Other scientists use similar techniques to try to create plants and animals unlike any ever found on earth.

When David succeeds, you'll find his squash in the supermarket. It will look like any other yellow crookneck squash. But you won't know that it's one of David's successes.

The government says it doesn't have to be labeled.

Randy Hampshire likes to talk about beans, and he likes to grow them, but he's had a hard time of it. His beans are organic, and he sells them, dried, in little one-pound plastic bags at the farmer's market: navy beans, black beans, kidney beans, chickpeas, Great Northerns, pintos. He'd have to sell an awful lot of beans to pay the bills for his farm.

As it is, he and his wife get up at three a.m. each Saturday to get ready for two farmers markets in suburban Detroit. It's nearly a three-hour drive each way. He mans a booth at one market, she tends a booth at the other. Both booths also offer home-baked breads, muffins, and other specialty items.

Sometimes they're home by four o'clock on Saturday afternoon.

"But I found out recently that I might be able to make a better profit by selling dried beans by the railroad carful—to the Japanese," Randy says. "The Japanese are willing to pay a real premium price for organic foods.

"We can't make a living trying to do it this way. Maybe we'll try it that way."

A colleague in his mid-twenties tells me that he never cooks for himself—he doesn't have time. Nor is he especially interested in cooking. In fact, he says with a small measure of pride in his voice, he's been so busy that he's eaten only meals from fast-food restaurants for more than three days running—breakfast, lunch, and dinner. It's good enough for him, he says.

Some weeks later he drops in to chat again. The doctor is telling him bad news about his health. His cholesterol is high, even his blood pressure is high. The doctor is puzzled, and so is he.

He is eating a triple-decker cheeseburger and an order of fries as he talks.

These stories are connected. I'd like to show you how.

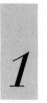

# *The Link Between the Farmer and Your Grocery Basket—and How It Is About to Change*

*The destiny of countries depends on the way they feed themselves.*

—Anthelme Brillat-Savarin,
nineteenth-century French gastronome-philosopher

*A*s the food editor of a metropolitan newspaper, part of my job is answering readers' questions about food safety and preparation. Most of the questions are simple: "How long is turkey good if it's kept in the freezer?" crops up every May, six months after Thanksgiving. Sometimes a reader really stumps me: "I have a can of tuna from my cupboard, and I have no idea how old it is. The sticker says it cost thirty-five cents. Is it still safe to eat?"

Still, I was unprepared for a reader who was puzzled by a recipe she'd read; it asked her to skin chicken breasts. Did this mean, she asked, that she was to peel the plastic film off the Styrofoam tray?

I was at first shocked by this ignorance. Didn't she know what chicken skin looked like? My next impulse was to laugh aloud—although I didn't. But her question troubled me. That reader simply had no connection in her mind between the pallid, essentially flavorless flesh she buys and the living, breathing creature from which it comes. She can't be faulted, nor can anyone who simply does not know how their food is produced: we have strayed so very far from the farm lanes and pastures whence our food comes.

A hundred years ago most Americans lived on farms or had friends or family who did. We knew that fruits and vegetables grew in their various seasons and what those seasons were. We understood that the beasts in the farmyard might end up on our tables; we were not squeamish about their deaths nor about our appetites.

In many ways the lives of our grandmothers and grandfathers on the farm were an ageless existence, not much different from the lives of their own ancestors. They did not have an easy time of it. Farm work was always exhausting and often frankly dangerous. As is true today, freak storms, droughts, floods, diseases, and pests that attacked stock and crop could destroy a year's work or worse. Calamities like fire, failed health, or a tough economy could drive a family from its land.

Still, the farm family lived out its years in the rhythm of the seasons. Winters were slow where winters were hard, but the duties of the farm were lighter at that time of year; the farmer's days were spent making repairs and tending to the stock. Spring brought the flurry of activity associated with new life and preparing the soil for seed; the long days of summer lent themselves to the unceasing work of raising crop and stock. By harvest time, the farmer and his family would be ready for winter's slower pace.

The men and women who worked the soil in those years were not concerned with making a profit nor with raising solely cash crops; they took their living from the land with the idea of feeding themselves and their children. We call such operations "subsistence farms" today, a phrase that wrongly suggests a bare hand-to-mouth existence.

But there aren't many of them left. There were 6.5 million farms in this country in 1917; today there are fewer than two million, and farmers represent less than three percent of our population. The Census Bureau announced in 1993 that it would no longer distinguish between "rural dwellers" and farmers; farmers are now "a statistically insignificant percentage of the population," the Census Bureau said.

But while the number of farms dwindled, the size of the remaining farms expanded; moreover, the number of people that each farm fed increased. This was due in part to advances in productivity made possible by new machinery, chemical fertilizers, pesticides, herbicides, hybrid seed breeding, and changes in livestock management. Science and technology brought new prosperity to agriculture.

The farmer who fed five or six people in 1917 would be stunned by his contemporary counterpart's achievement: the modern farmer feeds nearly a hundred people. And the farmer from 1917 would be stunned by another sight on a modern farm: the woman of the house usually buys her fresh and frozen food at the market in town like any urban dweller; she no longer grows, cans, and preserves against the winter.

As the number of farmers has decreased, it is hardly surprising that fewer and fewer of us have any working knowledge of the farm and its contributions, both social and economic, to our society. Farmers often complain that "the public" doesn't understand the farm's needs, and they are right: most Americans know no one who wrests a livelihood from the soil.

Nor does the public understand why food prices—prices that are the lowest of any industrialized country in the world—are so high at the supermarket. This perplexes the farmer, too. He knows that his share of the prices we pay at the store has actually dropped since World War II. In 1950, he earned about 36¢ on pork that sold for 53¢ a pound—a return of 67%. By 1993, the USDA's Economic Research Service reported, the farmer earned 72.5¢ on the pork that cost us $1.98 a pound; his share had dropped to 37%. While acknowledging occasional market price rises, a USDA agricultural economist said that the trend in the farmer's share of prices has been steadily downward. And in October 1994, when pork prices were at a 20-year record low, the farmer's return on pork had plummeted to 26%. He earned 50¢ of the $3.69 per pound I paid for pork chops. The key to the survival of the modern farmer has not been profit but productivity: at those prices he can compete only if he produces more.

Perhaps most important, because we have lost our connection to the farm, we have lost, too, our understanding of how and why our food is produced in the manner it is.

This can lead us to some ludicrous conclusions.

A survey of consumer attitudes on bioengineered foods conducted by assistant professor Thomas Hoban of North Carolina State University turned up this wryly amusing notion: "Consumers understand that food comes from the grocery store." Food, of course, *doesn't* come from the grocery store. It comes from the earth, in its essential origins.

Ironically, the shopper who thinks food comes from the grocery store wants to know more about how food is produced and how it ends up in the forms in which she buys it. She wants to know because food pervades the cultural, ethical, and spiritual dimensions of our lives. Food is so basic that anthropologists say humans seek shelter first, then food, and only then, when those crucial needs are met, does our species begin to think of sex.

For all of us food is also imbued with additional values: the aroma of a basil-strewn salad may remind an Italian-

American of his childhood in Boston's North End, which in turn may remind him of seeing his grandmother create that dish for his pleasure. The dishes we knew as children, those prepared by our mother's hands, are invariably those we want most when we are sick or tired or frightened.

Because food is so important to us on so many levels, we must generally trust blindly in government's promises of a safe food supply and in the safe practices of those who produce the foods we buy. We wade doggedly through complicated, confusing, and often contradictory information about the foods we eat. The reason is that most of us realize on a fundamental level that food choice is one of the last arenas in which we have some measure of control.

Yet trying to track where our food comes from is challenging. Each year more than 25,000 new products are introduced in American supermarkets, joining or replacing the 100,000 already in stock; few new products are truly new but are instead "product line extensions": new flavors of soft drinks and juices, new heat-and-eat concoctions, new spins on labor- and time-saving processed foods. Most push an existing product off the shelf. In the heavily competitive supermarket industry, where profit margins are a slim one percent, only products that sell will survive the continuous winnowing.

These products are called "value-added" foods, and it's easy to see why. The difference between the price of the corn in a box of cereal and the price we pay is the manufacturer's profit plus the costs of transportation from factory to warehouse to store, a food distributor's share of the proceeds, and the store's own markup. Every time a foodstuff passes through another set of hands, a few more pennies are tacked on to the price. We shoppers pay for those profits.

In 1973 we spent twenty-one cents of every food dollar for value-added foods ranging from jam to frozen dinners and meals eaten away from home. By 1987 that had risen to forty-one cents of every food dollar; some grocery industry analysts predict that by the year 2000, we'll spend ninety cents of every food dollar on foods prepared by strangers' hands.

We justify our willingness to spend our grocery money this way by asserting that we haven't time any more to cook, that our family's schedules are too hectic and mismatched to sit down to any meal, let alone one meal a day, together. If time is money, we say, then money is also time. We'll gladly spend money to buy ourselves a little time, time we desperately need in already overcrowded days.

### WHOSE VALUES ARE ADDED TO OUR FOOD?

"Value-added" is a term with many tiers of meaning. In its strictest business sense, it means that a manufacturer has added value to a raw ingredient by manipulating, processing, or some other tinkering. It is traditionally the manufacturer of the value-added product who gains respect and status. Calvin Klein, the fashion designer, has status (and so, we hope, will we if we buy his clothes), not the weaver whose machines produced the fabric used in the clothing, nor the spinner whose skills made the wool into yarn for the weaver, nor the shepherd whose sheep provided the wool for the spinner. It is diamond cutters and diamond setters who earn our admiration, not the sweat-shiny South African miners who pull those rough crystals from the ground for DeBeers's profit. Farmers, like miners, no longer have status in our society; they get little respect.

"Value" has another meaning: a principle or goal that a society supports. We speak of "family values" and of "core values." We wonder whether network television's prime-time programming is too violent for family values, and we might also wonder whether our values encourage violence. We agree easily that money and cost are two key values in our society—"You get what you pay for" stands against retailers' promises of "quality for less (money)"—although we sometimes grumble that society is too money-minded.

But money commands, in truth, a lesser value in our lives than other, profound commitments. We mean to stand fast with our families; that is a deep commitment and a solid value, sometimes prompting us to spend less time at work so we can nurture what we cherish. We express the value we invest in our community whenever we give time to youth groups, church activities, or charity work. We increasingly act on our commitment to the earth by placing a high value on recycling and on earth-friendly products—such a high value that in 1992 we spent $110.1 billion on products perceived to be eco-safe; gross sales of such products in 1993 were expected to rise to $121.5 billion.

Yet it is an almost universal human truth that we do not value what comes easily or is easily come by. Considering that America's food costs are so low, it's easy to understand the staggering waste of food we see in this country. A professor at the University of Arizona in Tucson used to conduct sociological research by having his students analyze garbage left out on Tucson's curbs for pickup. The students found all manner of perfectly good food—steaks, containers of yogurt, bread—in the garbage, together with wrappings and packaging of already prepared foods. Some social service agencies feed the hungry with food "rescued" from restaurant and institutional kitchens, carefully prepared food that otherwise would be thrown out because of a slow day or, perhaps, bad planning. And food banks salvage food to be discarded by manufacturers because of a misprint on the label or for other similarly silly reasons.

Cheap food makes its waste a guiltless act. We feel no

remorse when we toss out half-eaten or untouched foodstuffs that we allowed to spoil, because food is cheap and what is cheap has little value to us. Yet the city of Burlington, Vermont, discovered that about ten percent of its solid waste—garbage that its 40,000-odd residents paid to have trucked away to already bulging landfills—is compostable food scraps; the city has instituted methods to recover that waste as a compostable resource for community gardens.

When we treat food without respect because it is valueless, we lose our connection to our community—to the men and women whose toil produced it—and to the good earth that sustains us.

## CONSUMER OR CHOICEMAKER?

These concerns are not, I think, what the average shopper has on her mind as she mulls over dinner options.

She is thinking, instead, of how to feed her hungry family efficiently and easily. She may worry about a budget and whether there's money to go out to dinner or to splurge on steaks; she may also think about nutrition, hoping that the microwavable dinners stashed in the freezer will provide the vitamins her children need.

When she reaches the cash register, however, her purchasing decisions reflect her values.

A television advertising campaign mounted by McDonald's in 1994 depicted a harried mother flogging herself because she wasn't more like her own stay-at-home, June Cleaver mother: she didn't have dinner ready. When her two sons pointed out, quite sensibly, that she was not her mother but *their* mother, an expression of relief and delight washed over the young woman's face. Many loving hugs were exchanged. They celebrated her epiphany, of course, by rushing off to the neighborhood McDonald's for dinner.

Here is how that single decision reflects the fictional young mother's values, as explained by Michael Redcliff in *Sustainable Development: Exploring the Contradictions* (Methuen University Paperbacks, 1987):

> In the last 25 years, more than a quarter of Central America's rainforest has been turned to grass, and almost all the beef produced on it has gone to American hamburger chains. In 1960, the U.S. hardly imported any beef at all. By 1981, 800,000 tons were being imported at a price less than half that obtained in the U.S. As a recent article in the journal *Environment* put it: "The average domestic cat in the U.S. now consumes more beef than the average Central American."

I believe the fictional mother would be mortified to realize that she is, by her own example, teaching her sons that their wish for cheap hamburgers justifies destroying great swaths of the rain forest. Yet that is what she agreed to when she decided to patronize the family's favorite fast-food burger outlet.

The key phrase is "agreed to."

We have grown used to hearing ourselves described as consumers by every government and academic study that tracks economic progress and decline, by advertising and marketing surveys, by media reports. We use the word "consumer" to describe ourselves without stopping to think about what the word means:[1] to consume, to eat what is in front of you. Consuming is an essentially passive act; it suggests that the consumer has no choice in what he consumes. But we do

---

[1] A tip of the hat to Joe Domingues and Vicki Robin, whose excellent book *Your Money or Your Life* (Viking, 1992) amplifies this concept.

have choices, and that is why I have come to dislike being labeled a consumer. We make our choices, announce them
loud and clear, every time we buy an item: we vote with our
dollar, and we especially vote with our dollars at the supermarket. We control the marketplace and its offerings by buying—or *not* buying. That is why I think of myself, as I wheel
the wire buggy up and down the supermarket aisles, as a
choicemaker—every time I pluck a product off the shelf,
I *choose* to support the values and systems that lie behind
its production.

To make that choice, however, I have to understand the
values inherent in what I'm buying. Suppose that I live in
New York and I am considering buying some fresh broccoli
for my supper. I will think, quite probably, that this bunch of
fresh broccoli is superior to the stuff over in the freezer section. I will think that I have made a sound decision on my
family's behalf and think little more about it.

Yet here is A. V. Krebs in *The Corporate Reapers: The
Book of Agribusiness* (Essential Books, 1992) with some
thoughts on my broccoli purchase:

> Beyond the farm, the packaging and transportation
> of farm products consume enormous amounts of fuel.
> In the shift from home-cooked to mass-prepared
> convenience foods, energy costs have skyrocketed.
> Sugar gets refined; grains are milled and baked; oil-
> bearing seeds are crushed and refined; and fruits and
> vegetables are canned, dried or frozen. Such changes
> require massive amounts of steel, glass, aluminum
> and plastic.

But I'm buying *fresh* broccoli, so I don't have to think
about those things, right? Think again, says Krebs.

In 1984, New York area residents bought 24,000 tons of broccoli, most of it coming from California—2,700 miles away, at a transportation cost of $6 million. Hauling the refrigerated vegetable that distance also caused it to lose 19 percent of its vitamin C in 24 hours, 34 percent in two days. That same broccoli, which prefers cool growing weather, could have been produced in New York, not only saving Empire State residents transportation costs but also providing additional jobs and income for New York residents.

Now here is a dilemma. I do not favor all those energy costs involved in transforming fresh broccoli into a canned or frozen or further-processed vegetable. Neither do I favor the staggering energy costs involved in shipping fresh broccoli from California to New York—especially when its nutritional value deteriorates in the process. Is the answer to simply stop buying broccoli?

Perhaps. Or perhaps there are other solutions.

We are at a crossroads as a country and a culture, and many of the food-related issues of the future will depend on the decisions we make today.

## PLACING OUR TRUST IN SCIENCE

Canned foods, which we take for granted today, attained widespread availability and familiarity immediately after the Civil War. Companies that had perfected the safety and techniques of commercial canning during the war began to distribute their products nationally. That was, arguably, the beginning of the processed food industry, although milled flours and other value-added foods had been around long before.

Soon afterward, national advertising began to be a force in determining which products would succeed. Often advertising relied on the claims of scientific advances for credibility; the public began to trust in the claims that science made for new advances in food processing. We trusted that these new foods were safe and wholesome because science said they were. Advertising campaigns touted this reassuring science, hinting at the same time that there was status in buying and eating these "new and improved" foods.

But sometimes what science has given us has not proved to be as innocent as science claimed at first, as further research has revealed aspects of these new foods not previously suspected.

Consider the cholesterol concerns that swept the country in the late '70s and early '80s.

Learning that a diet high in cholesterol is linked to increases in heart ailments, we stopped buying butter. Instead, we spent our food dollar on margarine touted as cholesterol-free—only to be told, a few years later, that the process used to make margarine solid at room temperature, to resemble the butter we surrendered so reluctantly, may be worse for us than the butter itself. The jury is still out on trans-fatty acids, the culprits in hard margarines, but the miracle of cholesterol-free healthful margarine sticks seems badly tarnished by what we have learned since that miracle was introduced.

Today we face even more complex decisions about how we wish to feed ourselves and how we want to see food produced in this country.

Chief among these is whether to support genetically engineered foods—ranging from the Cal-Gene tomato, which has a relatively minor change in its DNA, to bovine somatotropin, the highly controversial hormone approved late in 1993 by the FDA for use on dairy cows.

These foods rely on sophisticated manipulation of the

chromosomes and genes of plants and animals; the resulting creatures may be patented by their developers, which guarantees both ownership and future profits. The moral and ethical issues surrounding the patenting of animal life were first brought to wide public attention when the Dow Chemical Company was awarded a patent in 1987 for its OncoMouse, a mouse whose genetic structure was altered to more closely mimic a human's, making it a better model for cancer research. But the issue had been settled, legally at least, some eight years earlier, when a scientist for General Electric named Ananda Mohan Chakrabarty won a patent for an oil-eating bacterium he developed through genetic engineering. GE hoped to market the bacterium as an aid in cleaning up oil spills like the *Exxon Valdez* spill in Alaska; GE later decided not to sell the fragile bacterium, which was too delicate to survive in the pounding seas.

Hundreds, if not thousands, of bioengineered foods now await government approval before they may be released. It looks like the government—in the guise of the Food and Drug Administration—will look kindly on them. In 1993 the FDA announced that it does not consider DNA a food additive, so these bioengineered foods will not need the agency's approval unless the foods contain a gene that might not be expected to be there normally. An example might be a tomato bioengineered to include a peanut gene; the Environmental Defense Fund and others have expressed concerns that such a tomato may pose a danger to a person who has a potent allergy to peanuts. Some researchers say one in twenty children suffers from food allergies; most of those seem to disappear as the child grows, but as many as two in a hundred adults have a violent allergic reaction to foods.

A visit to the labs where bioengineering research is ongoing might turn up carp, catfish, or trout with human genes incorporated to make them reach maturity—and market weight—faster; the visitor might see plants with flounder genes imported to give the plants more frost tolerance. Scientists in Canada have tried adding chicken and cow growth hormones to salmon in hopes of upping the fish's body size, and researchers have succeeded in bioengineering a salmon that is thirty-seven times larger than its naturally occurring counterpart. Experiments at the University of California at San Diego have succeeded in producing tobacco plants that glow night and day thanks to their firefly DNA; the technology could be transferred to other crops to permit night harvesting. Ohio State University researcher J. Mintz has foreseen development of cattle weighing more than 10,000 pounds and pigs that are twelve feet long and five feet tall, reports Dr. Michael W. Fox, vice president of the Humane Society of the United States.

In fact, an international market research firm called Frost & Sullivan predicted in 1989 that by the year 2015 all the chicken sold in the United States would be transgenic—that is, it would include genetic material from other species. While scientists acknowledge that poultry research is more difficult than such experiments on mammals—they have to figure out a way to manipulate embryos that are inside eggs, inside hens—they continue to work on disease resistance, better feed-to-meat conversion ratios, and faster growth to market weight. Frost & Sullivan also predicted that transgenic swine "should be on the market in seven to nine years"—by 1996, in other words—"and could take as much as half of the $10 billion U.S. market within the ensuing decade. Annual revenues to animal biotechnology companies would reach an estimated $150 million from U.S. sales and close to $500 million worldwide."

The research *is* expensive and has been going on for decades in corporate, university and government laboratories, funded with both public and private money. Dr. Vernon Pursel and his researchers at the United States Department of Agriculture's labs in Beltsville, Maryland, succeeded in creating Pig No. 6707,[2] which had human genetic material inserted in its DNA while it was still an embryo. Pursel hoped to cause the pig to grow faster and bigger and to produce leaner meat than it could have had it relied on its normal pig growth genes. They were successful, after a manner of speaking: the pig survived the manipulation and grew to adulthood. But Pig No. 6707 is covered with unusually long hair, is lethargic, probably sterile, and so arthritic that the beast can't stand up. This is unfortunate, say the scientists, who were hoping for a more productive outcome. Indeed, said Frost & Sullivan, "the very high value of the products means that 'secondary' effects such as *failure to thrive* can be ignored" (italics added). Translated, that means that it doesn't matter if the animals don't have much of a life; their value is in the price they'll bring at the market.

Pursel's experiments were prompted by the astonishing success of University of Pennsylvania researcher Dr. Ralph Brinster, who in 1982 thrilled the science community with proof that he had genetically engineered a supermouse that had human growth hormone in its DNA and could pass the improvement on to its offspring.

If the first bioengineered foods reaching the market are well received by shoppers, then industry will consider research to develop even more bioengineered foods a sound investment. But if the public does not embrace these foods, then industry may not pursue further research.

And industry already clamors for its share of biotechnology profits around the world. Australia has issued the first

[2]For further details on this research, see *The Human Body Shop* by Andrew Kimbrell (HarperCollins, 1993) and *Superpigs and Wondercorn* by Dr. Michael W. Fox (Lyons & Burford, 1992).

patent on a transgenic pig, a beast apparently similar to Pig
No. 6707 with added growth hormones to make it fatten
faster, and that pig's offspring are long past the seventh generation now. Pharmaceutical giant Merck & Co., Inc. applied
to the European Economic Community's Patent Office for exclusive rights to a "transgenic fowl expressing bovine growth
hormone," an application that drew fierce protest by animal
rights groups and social activists and has since been with-
drawn. Hundreds, if not thousands, of other similar patents
are still pending, both here and abroad.

Industry's rush to obtain approval is fueled by need. The
industrial style of agriculture we have practiced in this country since the end of World War II has led to its own set of
problems, as we shall see. When then–Secretary of Agriculture
Earl Butz said to farmers in the 1970s, "Get big or get out,"
he meant that factory ideals like efficiency, high-volume production, and standardization had to be adopted for farmers to
survive. And indeed, many farmers weren't able to compete.

Bioengineering sets out to solve problems that arise in
our industrial model of agriculture. The battery rearing of
chickens, keeping hundreds of laying hens in cages so closely
packed that the birds can barely move, is one way to make
the poultry raiser's job easier: all his birds are easily fed and
watered, and his time is used efficiently. But such close confinement stresses the chickens almost beyond their tolerance;
the result is that the chicks must be debeaked—that is, they
must have the points of their beaks nipped off—at early ages
so they won't peck each other to death. Diseases like avian
influenza, which rage like a brushfire in the crowded sheds,
can wipe out a farmer's investment in a matter of days.

It is certainly easier for a farmer to plow and plant
"hedgerow to hedgerow" as Butz encouraged; it is also easier
to plant a hundred acres of a single crop than it is to manage
the diverse needs of dozens of crops on that same land. But

the monocrop field looks like a smorgasbord to marauding pests, so the farmer must spray more and more pesticides as the insects and diseases adapt to his weapons. Planting the same crop year after year on the same land depletes the soil, so the farmer must use even higher rations of petroleum-gobbling manufactured fertilizers.

The logic of the bioengineering advocates is easy to follow. Why not use this technology, they say, to create chickens that are more resistant to disease and less afflicted by the stresses of close confinement? In this way, fewer antibiotics would be necessary, reducing the farmer's costs and improving the quality of the meat at the market. Why not create pigs that need less feed to grow to market weight, whose flesh is leaner, whose carcasses yield more marketable meat? Why not use this technology to produce squashes that are disease-resistant by "vaccinating" them at the genetic level? Why not produce tomatoes that won't suffer in a freeze; why not come up with hybrid breeds of corn that have a natural insect repellent in their genetic makeup?

All those ideas are in research and development, if not already nearing market release. And these ideas, together with the full range of other bioengineered crops and livestock being born in research laboratories, are aimed at solving the problems that come with the industrial model of agriculture.

The public is often leery of these ideas, and the scientific community doesn't always understand why. Scientists who research these new foods view the public warily because scientists think we are ill informed about the aims and possibilities that bioengineered foods represent. They believe, probably wrongly, that the technologies and principles involved in food bioengineering are too complex for the public to understand. ("Most of the fundamental ideas of science are essentially simple, and may, as a rule, be expressed in a language comprehensible to everyone," said Albert Einstein in *The Evolution of Physics.*)

At a 1993 industry-sponsored symposium on bioengineered foods in Washington, D.C., nearly every speaker mentioned Steven Spielberg's thriller *Jurassic Park*, based on the novel of the same name by Michael Crichton; all agreed that it might have given rise to public panic about the technological advances scientists consider possible through genetic manipulation. Spielberg's movie had other scientists concerned, too. "I worry that *Jurassic Park* may affect people the way another film, *The China Syndrome*, swayed public opinion against nuclear power," wrote biotechnology researcher Leroy E. Hood in an essay published in *The Detroit News* in the summer of 1993. "Will *Jurassic Park* set off a backlash against genetic engineering?"

They are concerned because bioengineering supporters believe this technology is simply a logical outgrowth of traditional agricultural practices like hybridization and crossbreeding. No one was alarmed when horses were crossed with donkeys to make mules, bioengineers argue; consumers accepted the broccoflower, a conventional cross of cauliflower and broccoli, quickly and enthusiastically. Transferring genetic material from one species to another is a natural next step, made possible by our increased knowledge and technological powers. They argue that these foods are the most tested products ever created in this country's history, and that they are perfectly safe to eat. They remind us that Thomas Jefferson panicked his neighbors by eating tomatoes at Monticello when everyone "knew" they were poisonous. They point to the public outcry raised against pasteurization when it was introduced at the turn of the century, a process reviled at the time as dangerous meddling with nature. They recall that Clarence Birdseye was ridiculed when he sought to introduce the first frozen foods.

Finally, bioengineering proponents are frustrated by the public's seemingly intentional misunderstanding of their purposes. Their goals are noble, they say: bioengineered crops may help end world hunger, may provide a bountiful crop where none has grown before.

The industrial model of agriculture works fine, say the bioengineering proponents, and the application of science can provide the fine-tuning to make it work even better.

But others say our industrial model of agriculture has had startling costs and that the luxury of cheap food has concealed the true cost of food production.

The chemicals used in agriculture are the leading polluters of our country's ground and surface water, dirtying half the country's watersheds and wells. Agricultural pollution is greater than all municipal and industrial sources of pollution combined. Particularly in the West, agribusiness is the largest user of publicly subsidized water for irrigation, water that comes from ancient, unreplenishable aquifers. Estimates of federal water subsidies paid from taxpayers' pockets to growers of animal feed range from $500 million to $1 billion each year.

In 1993 the state of North Carolina acknowledged that its major source of toxic waste was not a Superfund cleanup site but the swelling numbers of pigs raised in that state. Livestock produces 230,000 pounds of excrement per *second* in the United States; a feedlot of 10,000 cattle—or an intensive farm with 1,100 hogs—produces the same amount of waste as a city of 110,000 people. Runoff from the barns where those pigs are housed has fouled waterways and watersheds; it has made the water in neighbors' wells undrinkable.

Since farmers no longer aim to build the soil but hope to draw out of it in production only what they have put into it in the form of chemical fertilizers, the nation's topsoil is blowing away at astonishing rates. The USDA's Soil Conservation Service puts this loss at more than five billion tons each year; more than a third of the land in this country suited for agriculture has been lost to soil erosion.

The insects and diseases that farmers struggle to defeat have evolved into resistant forms, and they are no longer so easily destroyed; the chemicals that worked in low doses just a year before no longer work at all, even in higher doses. Pesticide use has seen a 3,300 percent increase since 1945, when petrochemical agriculture became the norm, yet crop losses due to insects have risen 20 percent in that same period. Despite DDT and a full spectrum of organophosphate pesticides, we have not eliminated a single species of pest.

Some 80 percent of all livestock and poultry raised in the United States receive antibiotics during their lives; more than half the antibiotics used in this country are given to livestock. The antibiotics used as feed supplements for chicken, pork, and beef, administered in "subtherapeutic" or low-level doses to help them grow faster, have spread through the human population. The result is that many diseases are now immune to the antibiotics doctors have available to treat them.[3]

"To say that chemical farming is efficient is to ignore the topsoil turning to hardpan, the ground levels collapsing above mined-out aquifers, the white salts glistening on the land," writes Paul Hawken in *The Ecology of Commerce: A Declaration of Sustainability* (HarperBusiness, 1993). "The most truly efficient farm is one that most effectively internalizes all of its costs. This is a farm that builds up topsoil, that uses water sparingly and thriftily, that uses pesticides rarely if at all, that understands that the secret to healthy plants is healthy soil, not deadly chemicals."

---

[3]See *The Antibiotic Paradox: How Miracle Drugs Are Destroying the Miracle* by Stuart B. Levy, M.D. (Plenum, 1992).

## MAKING ALLIES OF SCIENCE AND SUSTAINABILITY

The practices that Hawken mentions come under the heading of "sustainable agriculture," and its principles are simple. It mimics nature, rather than attempting to dominate it; it uses science to enhance, not displace, indigenous knowledge; it uses sun power, not petroleum power; it is nontoxic, as Hawken says, because it uses no pesticides or herbicides; it conserves topsoil and produces no off-farm impact; it recaptures and recycles all organic waste; it integrates livestock in a holistic system of farming; it treats livestock humanely; and it explores the links among healthy soil, healthy crops, healthy livestock, and healthy humans.

Sustainable agriculture practices—which include, but are not limited to, organic approaches—turn away from the aims of efficiency and higher production. Those who support sustainable agriculture cannot in good conscience endorse bioengineering of crops and livestock, they say, because they do not support the foundation of industrial thinking from which bioengineering springs. They see a large role for science in their style of agriculture, but not the kind of science that would manipulate the basic gene stock of existing plants and animals.

Sustainable agriculture supporters say they fear bioengineered varieties of seed and beast will drive out the ancient, slowly evolved varieties that humans have counted upon to feed themselves since antiquity. When a company like Upjohn can patent a plant—and own all rights to its use, demanding payment from anyone who wishes to plant it—the traditional wealth of the world's food sources is concentrated into fewer and fewer hands. What lies ahead, they ask, if corporations are able to patent cows and pigs and chickens and sheep, as seems likely when transgenic research becomes even more efficient?

The path of sustainable agriculture has many benefits, say its supporters, including more producers on smaller farms, who grow a more diverse variety of crops and live-stock. That is important for many noble reasons, they say, not the least of which is that it helps protect against a tragedy like the Irish potato famine, which began with the failed harvest of 1845. Even after the deaths of millions, the famine's effects lingered long afterward: widespread blindness due to malnutrition befell famine survivors. The potato famine was caused in part by a plant blight that killed the entire crop of potatoes in a country of smallhold tenant farmers—who all grew the same variety of potato, from seed purchased from their British landlords.

Advocates of sustainable agriculture argue that any man or woman who wishes to take a living from the land should be allowed—encouraged—to do so, something that is scarcely possible when agribusiness is a smallhold farmer's chief competitor. They say that their methods can feed as many people, if not more, as our current industrial methods.

And, they say, their ideals embrace the land and its culture; that will in turn help us embrace our own culture. Rural economies devastated in the farm financial crisis of the '80s could rise again; country towns can become lively, active, healthy assets if they are entwined with a system of small-hold farms.

As you will see, proponents of sustainable agriculture have a long way to go to see fair and equal treatment. As the regulations are now written, organic growers can't obtain crop insurance from the government. Because their crops are raised without the chemical inputs that conventional farmers use, organic growers are seen as bad risks. In some states, people who purchase their groceries with food stamps may not use them to buy produce at farmers markets or directly from a farmer. In most parts of this country the crucial "infrastructure" of processing plants for dairy farmers and supply lines for getting farm products to market in cities has long since disappeared. Meatpacking plants owned by transnational corporations have driven out of business or bought out their small, locally owned competitors.

## *WHO WILL FEED YOU IN THE FUTURE?*

In this book you will visit three kinds of farms: produce, dairy, and meat. You'll meet a farmer who produces his crops conventionally using industrially minded contemporary methods, who believes that bioengineering's promises will offer him a competitive edge. You'll also meet a farmer who raises his crops in a sustainable way, whose beliefs do not permit him to support bioengineered foods. Each of the farmers will talk about the values he brings to his work, why he does the things he does as he grows the food that is destined for your table. You will come to understand how your decisions at the supermarket or farmers market will affect each farmer, how you can vote in this important national debate.

And it is important. Here is Andrew Kimbrell, writing in *The Human Body Shop: The Engineering and Marketing of Life:*

> To a generation brought up with naive, techno-booster bromides—"Progress Is Our Middle Name," "Better Living Through Chemistry," "Cheap and Clean Nuclear Power," and even "DDT Is Good for Me"—the promises of utopian biotechnologists ring hollow. Certainly, for a society viewing a new genre of global environmental threats created by industrial pollution, it is now painfully evident that every

new technological revolution brings with it both benefits and costs. The more powerful the technology is at expropriating and controlling the forces of nature, the greater the disruption of our society and destruction of the ecosystems that sustain life. Society's experience with both the nuclear and petrochemical revolutions bears out this truth.

To fully understand the issues, it is important to frame the questions carefully, to be sure that you're asking the questions you need to have answered.

One question we won't ask is, "Which of these ways is the 'right' way to produce food in this country?" That question is unanswerable because the issues are complex. The people you will meet in this book have given those issues a great deal of thought, but they have reached different conclusions. All are well intentioned; there are no bad guys here.

Instead, you will want to ask: "Which of the ways in which food is produced most closely reflects my values? And what can I do to support those producers whose values and mine are most similar?"

The answers to these questions will come to you after you have visited the farms and heard the farmers speak.

So let's go. We have work to do.

# *A Lot of Technology in a Little Tomato*

*I*t is unseasonably cool on this overcast January day near the town of Immokalee in southwestern Florida, cool enough that Gary McKinsey wears an insulated vest and feels justified in a little good-natured grumbling about the weather. Gary is director of field production for Calgene Fresh, the company that would begin selling, as soon as the Food and Drug Administration permitted, a genetically engineered tomato under Calgene Fresh's MacGregor label. (The FDA approved Calgene's tomato for sale in the summer of 1994.) It is Gary's job to see that the fields where Calgene will plant these tomatoes are ready.

Gary is a bluff, hearty man in his forties; he wears his short dark hair combed back from his forehead and a pair of discreetly stylish aviator glasses. His handshake is firm, his manner open and friendly; he is the son of a Salinas Valley produce grower, and tomatoes are what he knows. Until June 1993, when he joined Calgene Fresh, Gary had spent his career in a part of the tomato industry called "gas greens"; there, volume is everything, he says, and he grew tired of that emphasis.

There are two ways of getting tomatoes to market in this country. In the gas-green method, the tomatoes are picked while they are still hard, far from ripe. From the fields, the tomatoes are delivered to a packer, who puts the still-green fruit in cardboard boxes of twenty-five pounds each. The tomatoes are sent to "degreening," a process in which they may spend three to five days in a sealed room filled with ethylene gas, to hasten their ripening. Then the newly colored tomatoes, now showing the faintest beginnings of their red-ripe optimal color, will travel to repackers, companies that specialize in removing tomatoes from the 25-pound boxes and divvying them into smaller boxes of tomatoes that are all the same size and same color. These boxes are destined for shipment to chain-owned grocery produce buyers, produce markets or to produce brokers, who will sell them to smaller, independent grocery stores, wholesalers and restaurants and institutional kitchens at prisons, colleges and school-lunch programs.

The other way tomatoes are delivered in this country is the "vine-ripe" system. To the average shopper, "vine-ripened" is misleading; it is a United States Department of Agriculture term, and it applies to any tomato that has begun to show any color whatsoever before picking, no matter how little. It does not mean, however, that the tomato actually ripened on the vine, as the vine-ripened tomatoes we pluck from our backyard plants are allowed to do.

"Vine-ripes"—sometimes called "pinks" in the trade—follow most of the same steps along the way from field to market as gas-green tomatoes do. But because vine-ripes are more fragile, the speed in the packing house lines is slower, and the tomatoes are handled with a little more care. The key to success in the vine-ripe line is not necessarily volume but getting as many unbruised, undamaged fruits to market as possible.

Either way, the tomatoes are 10 days or more from the field by the time they get to your neighborhood store. Your grocery's produce manager wants the tomatoes to last at least four days after delivery so he'll have a chance to sell them to you and your neighbors.

None of this contributes to the arrival at market of a delicate, fully ripe tomato bursting with the kind of flavor we all wish tomatoes might have.

That, according to Calgene Fresh officials, is why they set out to grow and sell their genetically engineered tomato. The company's sales materials say the MacGregor tomato will have "summertime farm stand vine-ripened flavor." They chose the name MacGregor for their special line of tomatoes because focus groups found that name, of all the choices offered, the warmest and friendliest; it echoes, the groups said, Farmer McGregor, the farmer from the Peter Rabbit stories. (No one in the focus groups or in Calgene's marketing division, apparently, remembered that Farmer McGregor's chief accomplishment was killing Peter Rabbit's father and eating him "in one of Mrs. McGregor's pies.")

What the scientists in Calgene's labs discovered was a way to slow the ripening of a tomato. They learned how to make a copy of the gene that acts as the tomato's biological clock, if you will. This gene "tells" the tomato when to begin to soften and rot. It is, actually, in the tomato's interest to do so early. Rotting tomatoes split when they fall to the ground, giving their seeds a chance to be spread around. From the tomato's point of view, rotting is good: it hastens the spread of the species. But from man's point of view, rotting is, of course, bad: no shopper intentionally chooses an overripe, squishy tomato.

So the Calgene scientists learned how to turn off that gene, by inserting a copy of the same gene backward. The result is a tomato that "stays fresh longer," the company says; critics say it's yet another tomato that's engineered for the market, not for the shopper, and that the three or four extra days these tomatoes stay on the vine is not long enough to improve their flavor dramatically.

Calgene's bioengineered tomato is not a single variety, but a way to manipulate the genetic structure of any tomato, whatever its variety. Thus the company's plant breeders work to incorporate Calgene's patented bioengineering techniques into a number of commercial strains of tomatoes. Some people argue that these varieties will replace conventionally bred tomatoes—and, similarly, replace other kinds of crops. The critics say that eventually Calgene may control rights to almost all the tomatoes planted in this country, perhaps in the world.

Calgene has acquired a patent on this genetic technology, called an "antisense" gene; every other plant breeder and seedsman who wishes to avail himself of the technique to improve some other vegetable will have to pay Calgene a royalty. Calgene also will collect royalties on another gene it has patented, a gene which gives an organism resistance to an antibiotic called kanamyacin; scientists use that gene as a test to see if other bioengineered traits have been passed along in a plant as they had hoped.

But even without those royalties, there is big money in tomatoes.

We are virtually the only country in the world whose citizens have come to expect and demand tomatoes year-round. One could argue that it is our own stubborn disregard for the limits of seasonality that have brought us to this odd moment: The tomatoes we buy look like tomatoes, it is true, but they no longer taste like the tomatoes we remember. This is because tomatoes have been bred to be shipped thousands of miles without softening or spoiling, bred to stand up to mechanized harvesting and processing, bred to keep long enough that the produce manager in the corner grocery store can make his profit from them.

Other people profit, too. As John Seabrook explained in a July 1993 *New Yorker* article about Calgene's tomato, the men—and it is almost exclusively men—who distribute tomatoes in this country can make millions of dollars a year, millions of dollars earned by controlling the movement of tomatoes from field to market. "The longer the shelf life of a tomato, the greater the probability that all the people who speculate on tomatoes—salesmen, repackers, warehousers, and retailers—can sell them for more than they bought them for," wrote Seabrook. "The wholesale market is very large, and a lot of money is involved; the price of a twenty-five-pound box of tomatoes can move from six dollars to eighteen dollars in ten days."

All this is why Gary McKinsey has a job with Calgene Fresh.

Calgene Fresh hopes to capture just fifteen percent of the $23 billion winter tomato market—that is, tomatoes sold from October through June. In doing so, the company would earn $8 billion in the first year, quite a return on the estimated $20 million it has spent to develop this tomato. Calgene believes that most of its customers will be those who have quit buying substandard winter tomatoes; it believes its genetically engineered tomatoes will command a premium price, simply because of their perceived higher quality.

The 189 acres of sandy Florida soil that Gary visits on this cool, breezy January day will one day grow Calgene

Fresh's genetically engineered tomatoes. But for the moment, in a sort of dry run while the company awaits FDA approval for its genetically engineered tomato, the fields are being planted with conventional tomatoes, tomatoes whose DNA has not been manipulated in other than conventional methods. The field crews are planting two varieties widely grown in Florida, where most of the tomatoes sold east of the Mississippi in winter come from: Sunbeam and Agriset. They'll be ready to pick in about two months, the only crop that Florida's tough tropical climate will allow this year. Then other fields—in Alabama, Georgia, perhaps North Carolina, New Jersey, and Ohio—will be planted and picked in succession. The harvests move north as the summer wears on, until at last, when frost hits the northernmost, fields in Mexico will begin their harvest and will carry the market until the re-planted Florida fields bear fruit. Distribution systems are different in the West, where two crops a year can be grown in California; but fewer than two percent of California's tomato harvest makes it to market east of the Mississippi, Gary says. Since the energy crunch in the '70s, it isn't profitable to ship tomatoes so far.

Calgene Fresh has created its own distribution system for its specially handled, specially packed—and eventually, specially bred—tomatoes, a system unlike any other now in existence in this country. As each Calgene field is harvested in the seasonal succession, its crop is shipped to Calgene Fresh's distribution plant on the south side of Chicago; we'll visit there a little later. Calgene Fresh has established its own "vertically integrated" produce distribution system; the company controls everything about these tomatoes, from seed to store. It's an idea that Calgene has borrowed from both the poultry and swine industries, and it has many benefits for the company, but fewer for the producers, as we shall see.

In the field where Gary stands, the soil is light in texture and color; it's called "sugar sand," and the reason for the name becomes clear as soon as you pick up a handful. It's finer even than the kind of sand used to fill children's backyard sandboxes. All the Calgene fields in this area are ringed by levees and deep drainage ditches put in at tremendous expense, says Gary; they're required to protect the nearby waterways from chemical run-offs. Not far to the southwest stand the Everglades, but even here, with the water table just thirty-six inches below the ground, the land is delicate and vulnerable. On one side of the Calgene parcel is a citrus grove, its trees in the last stages of harvest: Immokalee is in the heart of the Florida citrus-growing region. On the other sides of the parcel, the vegetation looks wild and tropical, with swales of sawgrass, patches of palmetto, and live oak trees draped with the parasitic Spanish moss. The birds that populate the Everglades wheel and dance across the skies here, too: egrets flap lazily by, and kites patrol ceaselessly, looking for an easy meal. It's easy to believe that the land bides its time to reclaim these fields.

If this land wasn't used for tomatoes, says Gary, it would grow citrus or melons or squash; but it wouldn't grow anything of use to man if man didn't manage it.

And so the rows and rows of tomato seedlings are set into small berms of sugar sand covered with black plastic, partly to keep weeds down and partly to help warm the earth for the tender young plants' roots. A thousand pounds of chemical fertilizers are laid down on each acre over the course of the growing season, and Gary is proud when he says that he's monitored the fields so closely that he can report that only 15 percent of the fertilizer is lost to the soil and groundwater. Each plant needs a pound of nitrogen a day before it begins fruiting, he says with knowledge born of experience; after it sets fruit, it will need a pound and a half a day. The little plants grow well only with steady drip irrigation in

the beating, merciless sun and sterile soil, he says; they get an
inch of water every twelve hours, flowing at a rate of a half-
gallon per minute through the plastic pipelines laid into the
earth. The irrigation lines are set up to release water for two
hours, then shut off for two hours, says Gary; this prevents
the water from "welling" around the plants' roots, which
would push the sandy soil away from the plants. It is water
management, not higher applications of fertilizer, that make
nice, big tomatoes, Gary explains. Tomatoes grown on over-
watered plants grow very big—but suffer in shipping, the
antithesis of what a vine-ripe shipper wants.

Having grown up in the Salinas Valley, Gary is well-
versed in the mysteries of tomato growing; he knows what's
required to make every plant bear to its maximum potential.
And because he is affiliated with the University of California
at Davis's agricultural programs, he keeps current with new
approaches to plant culture. He talks about the difficulties of
convincing contract growers in Florida and Mexico—the
farmers who use their knowledge and equipment to grow
tomatoes on Calgene's land—to try doing things a new way.
There is a hint of belligerence in his voice when he says that
"they're growing these tomatoes for us, so they'll damned
well do it our way!" Gary wants these growers to use tools
such as beneficial insects released to prey on pests, rather
than spraying pesticides; he wants them to accustom themselves to fallowing, or resting, some of their fields every year
so the land can recover. He has introduced them to the notion
of planting cover crops between the rows of tomatoes so they
won't have to spray herbicides to keep weeds down. In addition, this will later improve the soil when the cover crops are
plowed in as "green manure." Gary is teaching them about "integrated pest management," which establishes some tolerance
for pests and disease and doesn't spray until those tolerances are
breached. Besides teaching these growers about the benefits

of lower "inputs," as Gary calls them, he also helps Calgene's growers understand the importance of monitoring "nutrient uptakes." The language of agriculture has shifted to a pseudotechnical jargon, so "inputs" are the chemicals used to produce a crop; "uptake" is how much of those chemicals the plants actually use. The higher the inputs, the more expensive it is for a grower to produce a crop; the less efficient the plants' uptakes, the more money the farmer wastes.

It's been difficult for Calgene to locate growers for their tomatoes, says Gary, because big packing firms control the market, and growers are bound by contract and custom to sell their tomatoes to the giant packers. These arrangements, which have become entrenched in just a few generations, are not always to the growers' benefit. The packing house puts up half the initial investment and the grower puts up the other half, but at the end of the season when the accounts are reckoned, the packer makes a number of deductions from the grower's profits. These include packing costs, gassing costs in the gas-green market, and "palletization" costs, that being a fee for stacking the boxes of tomatoes on pallets for easier shipment.

The two farmers who grow tomatoes for Calgene in Florida receive a monthly wage and incentives; Calgene owns the land, but these farmers may make up to $100,000 a season if all goes well, Gary says.

It's a high-stakes gamble based on a terribly fragile fruit.

"Remember, that's a living thing you're dealing with," says Gary. "Tomatoes keep living after they're picked. The stem-end is an open wound that is vulnerable to bacteria and spores in the air, as vulnerable as a cut on your finger. All the natural processes speed up after picking."

Furthermore, tomatoes ripen from the "shoulders"—the top of the fruit, near the stem end—down. They show color first on the shoulders, and indeed that's where graders look to judge their stage of ripening. Since the shoulders ripen first, that is also where the first signs that a tomato is past its prime appear: a slight wrinkling and drawing in of the skin. All this is why most of the pre-packed tomatoes we see in the grocery store are placed in their little fiberboard trays with their shoulders down: It's a deceit that packers and sellers practice on shoppers, and a good reason why you shouldn't buy tomatoes you can't inspect thoroughly.

Gary agrees to show us around the rest of the parcel, and we pile into his rented pickup truck. It's rented because Gary travels a lot: Between June 1992 and January 1993, he had logged more than a hundred thousand air miles, enough frequent-flier miles to keep him and his family in free tickets for the rest of the year. He misses his wife, his infant daughter, and the five-year-old son who is so clearly the light of his father's heart. But it will be some time before Gary's life settles into a more sedentary pace and he can spend time at home in Sacramento, California.

As we jostle around the perimeter of the fields, Gary explains what the contract crews of field hands—men and women, most with the blood of the Aztecs showing in their high, flat cheekbones and inky eyes—are doing. Some of these crews have come up from Mexico; a few have been recruited from local labor. Several plant seedlings by hand, a job which requires working along the plastic-covered rows while bent at the waist. We stop for a moment to watch a trio of young men work in a ballet of concentrated motion: They are tying seedlings planted earlier to stakes, and they have devised rudimentary tools to make their labor easier, more efficient. With two quick motions and an arcing of one tireless arm, looking like wizards waving magic wands, two of the men tie up the plants. The third follows, to snug any loose ends. Gary says the men in the fields often sing while they work, but they aren't singing today, at least not yet. They sing, he says, songs in a language that he doesn't understand: "songs about home, I guess."

The big tractor and planting rig that might ordinarily be used is bogging down in the soft slick soil in this part of the field, he explains, which is why the crew is planting by hand. We watch for a moment as the tractor, riding high on wheels set far apart to clear the carefully mounded berms, catches on some black plastic and tears it off the best part of a row. That plastic isn't reusable, Gary has said. It will be thrown away, and new stuff will have to be laid there. The back of the rig drawn by the tractor has two jutting seats for workers to sit on as they plant; those, too, are useless for the moment.

It's too bad, Gary says; the tractor and rig make things more efficient, easier for everyone. The rig automatically punches a hole in the black plastic for the seedling and another for the wooden stake which will come soon afterward. The crew members riding on the rig would settle the small plants into the soil with a deft two-fingered push-and-twist motion, and others would follow to firm the plants' footings.

The young grower whose responsibility these fields are has come twice to speak to Gary; he looks to be in his early thirties, and the skin around his eyes is drawn taut in an expression of constant worry. He and his family live on the grounds in a house that was part of the parcel when Calgene bought it. It's a handsome place, a two-story, generous-sized, cedar-sided house raised on stilts, as many houses hereabout seem to be. A brightly colored plastic tricycle and a swing set grace the oasis of a yard: there is at least one toddler in residence, it would appear. Laundry flaps in the cool breeze, and there are flowers planted here and there. The grower and his young family will stay in this house, Gary says, although this parcel will be fallowed next year and he will work another field nearby.

Gary's background gives him an affinity for the soil and

the land. When he talks about his Salinas Valley childhood, his voice softens a little, and he explains with carefully concealed regret that his father's land can support only his parents and his brother's family. So Gary had to go out into the world to find land to farm, and that is what he has found with Calgene. "We have to protect this," he says, stooping to pick up a handful of sugar sand. "They aren't making it anymore." His passion for the land is obvious—he doesn't immediately dust off his palms, as a city-dweller might—but it is a doomed passion, it would seem. Gary is pessimistic about whether the next generation in this country will have enough farmers to work the land: "There isn't any money in it anymore, it seems like," he says. Asked how he could interest his young son in farming, the son whose fearlessness and prowess have been at the center of most of his father's stories about him, Gary shrugs in painful eloquence. "If he wants to do that, I might try to discourage him," he says thoughtfully, "or maybe not. But I don't think he'll want to. What's in it for him? He'll see the brokers driving their expensive cars, with their gold and their Rolexes; why shouldn't he want that instead?"

We are silent for a moment. Gary studies the ground, his hands in the pockets of his jeans, his feet firmly planted and motionless, his hair barely riffling in the light snapping breeze. I have the sense that there is a broken heart hidden in this man, a sense that he buried a dream when he realized that he would have to leave his family's land. But I also sense that Gary is not a complainer and that those old griefs are long and deeply concealed.

I ask him what he might want if he could have anything in the world. This, only bigger, he says: "My dream? Some place three times this big, with three times the productivity, three times the volume."

I ask Gary what he thinks about sustainable agricultural

practices, and he sighs. He would love to reduce his inputs and protect the soil and the environment; that is part of the reason why he works so closely with the UC-Davis agricultural programs, and why he wrestles with stubborn growers to convince or coerce them to try new methods. But he doesn't think it can be done commercially and still feed us—the public who cries out for more and cheaper food. As an experiment back in California, he planted a patch of tomatoes that received no chemical inputs at all; he managed it organically and was rewarded with a beautiful crop. "But the second crop was completely destroyed," he says. "That second crop was lost to pests and disease—because it was later in the season, when both of those threats had reached their peaks." And that, Gary adds, is why commercial growers can't yet manage their farms in completely sustainable ways: we wouldn't have the winter salads we demand; there would be no lettuces, no tomatoes, no out-of-season produce. Moreover, a grower can't make enough money to survive on a single crop each year. No, it simply isn't possible for large-scale commercial growers to grow our food without using any chemicals at all, Gary says.

He offers to give us a tour of Immokalee, the town of about eleven thousand inhabitants where a good bit of Florida's gas-green tomato industry is centered. It is a surprisingly long drive, perhaps twenty minutes from the Calgene fields, a drive through acre after acre of citrus groves and beef pasture. The sandy soil isn't good for much else, Gary says again, although he is momentarily distracted by a realtor's sign on a street corner advertising some three hundred acres of "prime agricultural land" for sale. Looking it over with a practiced eye as we roll by, he says that Calgene might be looking for still more land in the area; that parcel may interest the company.

On the way to Immokalee, Gary drops out of the conversation in the truck for a moment to make a long-distance call on the cellular telephone that accompanies him everywhere. "I want to make a calling-card call to Mexico," he tells the international operator. From memory he reels off both his calling-card number and the number he's calling, that of one of the Calgene growers. He seems unamazed later when I remark on the wonder of calling a Mexican employee from a pickup truck traveling fifty miles an hour in rural Florida. A shrug says this is commonplace to him, although he confesses that the telephone bills he racks up are extraordinary.

He tells me that Immokalee is in Collier County, named for the family, he says with what sounds like a mixture of admiration and derision, that "owns it." Two packing houses for gas-green tomatoes in Immokalee are owned by Colliers, brothers or cousins who had some sort of a falling out; the local paper is owned by Colliers as well. And as we drive into town, we pass a local landing strip for small aircraft: a little private plane is just coming in, and Gary says he recognizes a man in the plane descending not fifty feet away as one of the packing-house Colliers.

The part of Immokalee we drive through as we enter the town is pretty in a south Florida way: the houses are mostly ranch-style, newer homes, almost all with five-foot-tall chain-link fences ringing their yards. Used to California real estate prices, Gary marvels at the affordability of land and houses around these parts.

For a stretch of about a mile, we pass packing house after packing house, some quartered in well-maintained, fairly new buildings of brick, others in much older, much more dilapidated frame buildings. Dotted among the plants on both sides of the street are small grocery stores, restaurants, and the kind of roadside bars that have no windows; most of them advertise specials or coming attractions with signs written only in Spanish.

Our progress through Immokalee is blocked by an overturned open-back truck of gargantuan proportion; the road is filled with thousands of hard green tomatoes, some of them still rolling about as we approach. I remark that the packer whose truck this is will feel quite a loss, and Gary laughs. "Hell, they could just scoop those things up and pack 'em anyway," he says, tongue in cheek, about the gas-green packers he has come to dislike so much. "They'll be bruised, but it won't matter much to those guys." He is kidding, of course; but I am surprised to see that few of the tomatoes are shattered or smashed. "They bounce," Gary says of the immature tomatoes. "They bruise, but they bounce. That's why they can run those packing lines so fast."

There is not much else for us to see in Immokalee, so Gary suggests that we stop for lunch on the way to the Fort Myers airport.

Over lunch Gary tells about growing up and how his parents used to come visit him when he was in college, bringing fifty-pound bags of dried beans, baskets of fresh produce, anything that would feed their hungry son and his friends. "Life was easy then," says Gary; he and his peers would fire up a barbecue and share the wealth. Everyone always shared what they had, so everyone was always fed; no one ever went hungry. Those were happy, happy days, he says.

Gary orders a Caesar salad with a grilled chicken breast—though we are at a beef house—and in doing so, tells me that he struggles with his weight these days. He tries to eat lightly while he's on the road, and he tries to stay fit by exercising whenever possible, but his schedule is grueling, and finding time is difficult. I hesitate and then decide that he probably doesn't want or need to know that the "diet" lunch he's just ordered probably has more fat and cholesterol— from the cheese and the egg-enriched salad dressing—than the thickest steak on the lunch menu.

■　　■　　■

Some twenty hours later, I am in Chicago, which is tentatively reemerging from a spate of record-breaking winter cold. Here in the vibrant, lively downtown area there are few pedestrians, and those who are out and about are muffled from their toes to the top of their heads. Anything goes in Chicago when the weather's like this, says a friend; it's almost a badge of pride to look goofy when you go out in this weather.

In a few moments, Calgene's Jeff Bergau will pick me up and we will visit the company's near–South Side distribution center. Jeff, a bright, cheery blond in his mid-twenties, has a master's degree in communications from Syracuse University. He, too, is a relative newcomer to Calgene Fresh, having left the public relations firm of Porter-Novelli, which handled the Calgene account. Jeff was with us in Florida and has said several times that he loves to visit Calgene's fields: "Sometimes it just makes me feel like I want to chuck it all and go work as a farmer. There is something about that life—working on the land, working out in the open air—that really appeals to me. You'd get away from all the pressures of the way we live today." Later, he tells me that his grandparents lived on a farm outside Chicago before they moved to the city; he remembers going there as a child. I wonder, but do not ask, why they left, and whether Jeff feels very far removed from the farm.

En route to the Calgene distribution center, Jeff, a vocally appreciative Chicago adoptee, says the center is quartered near the Pullman neighborhood. He describes the fights that went on to preserve this neighborhood, built by George M. Pullman, creator of the Pullman railroad sleeper car, as a national historic area. In the end the advocates won, he says, and the neighborhood was saved from the bulldozer. He tells this story with some appreciation, saying that he regrets our national tendency to pull down and bulldoze the old, only to replace it with a not-always-superior new.

But the area looks distinctly tired, and Chicago's status

as an aging industrial city seems unchallenged when you look around these grimy streets. The houses are set cheek-by-jowl; many are sided with asphalt shingles, and a lot of the porches sag wearily, as if they are as tired as their hard-working residents.

The neighborhood shifts as we draw nearer the distribution center, and the air is tinged with the faint aroma of rotting vegetables. It is an odd scent on this bitter-cold sunny day, one perhaps expected in near-tropical New Orleans, but not in a warehouse district in winter-bound Chicago.

Calgene Fresh is unusual in deciding to locate its distribution center here, Jeff says, where there are not many produce distributors. And, he adds, it is not certain that Calgene Fresh will ever open another distribution center elsewhere; the company is headquartered in nearby Evanston and is committed to the Chicago area. As of now the company thinks all its national distribution will be adequately served from here.

The distribution plant is quartered in a deceptively small-looking building in the bare-bones construction style favored in warehouse districts of today.

In the small foyer the two women at the reception desk greet Jeff by name; they chat, the three of them, about some pipes that froze in the recent hard weather. This is less business than office gossip, it seems: Jeff, to my knowledge, has nothing to do with insulation and buildings in this company. A four-foot-high potted corn plant, a *Dracena marginata*, sits in a corner by the stairs up to the statistics and accounting department; it is wilted and brown, obviously dead.

At each turn Jeff is a gracious host, introducing me promptly to everyone we meet. I notice that he always identifies me as a journalist, which serves as a gentle warning to those we'll speak with, and cues his coworkers so polite conversation may begin. The people I meet are warm and friendly without exception.

We walk through a large, clean, well-lit lunchroom where someone is heating up a lunch in the microwave, the savory smell filling the room. Again Jeff is greeted by name. Some of these men and women work in the packing room, and I am surprised that they know Jeff. He laughs, saying that he's worked on the packing line alongside some of them; it is Calgene Fresh's policy, part of the "core values" that Jeff often refers to but does not fully explain, that everyone in the company joins in whatever work must be done. On at least one occasion he worked a Saturday afternoon on the packing line next to Stephen Benoit, then Calgene Fresh's vice president for marketing and Jeff's immediate superior. "We weren't very good at it," he says affably, "but it was fun."

We begin the tour of the packing facilities in the cold-storage rooms. Here cardboard boxes of tomatoes stacked ten or so high rest on pallets, awaiting their turn to be moved into temperature-controlled ripening chambers. Calgene, being a vine-ripe company, doesn't gas its tomatoes, Jeff says; instead, it controls the tomatoes' coloring and ripening by raising and lowering the temperature. But it is not right to call these chambers "refrigerators," he says. They are never kept as cold as a refrigerator because refrigeration ruins a good tomato.

Some of the stacks of boxes of tomatoes have come from Calgene's own growers; others have arrived from growers who have sold their product to Calgene for packing. Until the FDA approved Calgene's bioengineered tomatoes early in 1994, all these tomatoes were conventionally bred varieties.

Now Jeff steers us past a bank of desks where workmen are installing more phone and computer lines. This is where the company's data processors will work, the folks who keep track of all manner of information, from the number of boxes packed to which employees worked when. The vast room has a two-story ceiling; it is slightly cool here but not unpleasantly so. While the machinery on the packing line is relatively noisy, conversation is possible at just a notch or so above normal volume.

The frequent beeping of forklifts backing up forms a backbeat for the syncopated rhythms of the packing lines. Forklifts deliver twenty-five-pound boxes of tomatoes to a fellow at the bottom of a slanted conveyor belt; he transfers the boxes to the belt, which carries them up to a man standing on an elevated platform perhaps fifteen feet above the floor. One by one, the man on the platform tips the boxes of tomatoes into a wide, shallow bed that rolls the tomatoes through a washing mechanism. Calgene Fresh doesn't wax its tomatoes as some packers do, says Jeff; its tomatoes get their gloss naturally in the wash-and-buff process.

The newly clean tomatoes roll some fifty feet farther, where they drop about a foot onto another line that will carry the fruit past graders who work on both sides of the line. The graders, about a dozen or so men and women, must work quickly: they pluck out any obviously damaged fruit and sort the rest by degree of color and ripeness. The best quality tomatoes will be packed for the premium-priced MacGregor's label; the second-tier quality will reach institutional and restaurant kitchens, where the fruit's appearance isn't as important as its slicing or cooking quality; and the lowest quality will be sold under a generic label.

The top-quality tomatoes are routed along the conveyor belt to a row of some fifteen men and women who sort, grade, and place the tomatoes into specially designed "packs"—the fiberboard separators that will hold the tomatoes safely in their boxes. Jeff tells me that these gray-brown cardboard packs are made from recycled paper and are themselves recyclable; they feature a little disk of airspace, about the size of a dime, at the bottom of each cup, which improves air circulation around the tomato and keeps its quality high, he says. Tomatoes of several different sizes and stages of ripeness are packed here; a sign above each work bay reminds the packer which kind he is packing that day.

The packers work at a less intense speed than the graders who preceded them on the line, but they are intent on their work nonetheless. There is little talking; eyes and hands stay directed on the work before them. They handle the tomatoes carefully, turning them this way and that to inspect for damage and blemishes; they pick through the tomatoes shunted to their work bays to match as closely as possible tomatoes of the same size and ripeness in the boxes they pack. Jeff says the line is running at about half its full-capability speed today. I say that the work must be numbing for the employees, but Jeff counters that the people on the lines wouldn't mind going faster. Everyone here works on his or her feet all day, except for breaks and meals, but I notice padded mats beneath the workers' feet, to cushion their feet and legs from the concrete floors. Jeff won't tell me exactly what the graders and packers are paid, but he does say that the fifty-odd employees earn "better than union wages."

The best-quality tomatoes will be sent through a labeling machine, where they'll have a little sticker applied to their stem, a MacGregor label. Calgene packs its brand-name tomatoes shoulders-up, not shoulders-down like the rest of the industry. "It's like we're packing with our pants down," says a Calgene salesman, who immediately looks as if he regrets the flip image. But I understand: shoulders-up means that shoppers will see the most vulnerable part of the tomato first so they'll be able to tell at a glance if the tomato is in its prime.

The MacGregor-labeled tomatoes are by now packed in one-layer flats, shallow cardboard boxes designed to stack one atop the next yet still leave plenty of air space between the boxes. Again, says Jeff, this is to preserve the quality of the tomatoes.

Jeff says the company has had no trouble finding buyers for these tomatoes in the competitive tomato trade. That's partly because the tomatoes come ready to display in their special flats; the produce manager at the market doesn't need to winnow through them to remove any damaged fruit, and he doesn't need to pay someone to stack them in loose displays.

Tomatoes that were graded as second quality, destined for food service use, get repacked in larger boxes, but they do not benefit from the special cardboard packs: they are simply tumbled into the boxes and weighed, each box averaging about twenty-five pounds. These tomatoes don't get the special stickers.

The third-level tomatoes are today being packed in four-tomato cellophane-overwrapped rectangular green fiberboard trays for special buyers; these tomatoes, which won't bear the MacGregor label either, are packed shoulders-down and will eventually appear at lower-end supermarkets, Jeff says.

Finally, the MacGregor-label tomatoes get one last looking over by still another employee whose job it is to catch any blemished or bruised tomatoes before they leave the plant. He may remove some tomatoes from a flat, consolidating flats as necessary so that every tomato in a flat is the same shade of red, the same size, the same-same-same—that's what the supermarket buyers want, Jeff says.

We look over a flat that holds MacGregor-labeled tomatoes as big as softballs. Jeff says this is the size produce buyers *think* the public wants, although Calgene's market research says shoppers actually want smaller tomatoes, the size of, say, a tennis ball. I second that research; the smaller tomatoes look more "right" to my eye, the size for a salad for two or a couple of sandwiches.

Now the finished flats are stacked for ease of loading on

the trucks that will deliver them. They are beautifully appealing, these tomatoes. They have a lovely color and just the
right heft in the hand, a heft that promises lots of flesh, not
much watery juice.

Remember, though: these are simply conventional tomatoes, carefully handled. These are not yet Calgene's bioengineered tomatoes.

Still, I have to remind my cook's hand not to dart into a
box and pluck one of these beauties up, up to my mouth.
They look good on such a cold, cold day. It has been a long
time since summer, since I picked ripe tomatoes in my garden. It would be easy to succumb to the desire, to justify a
tomato in the dead of winter simply because I remember how
good a tomato in its season can be.

I am, it would seem, exactly the kind of customer that
Calgene Fresh wants: a shopper who has lost faith in winter
tomatoes but who cannot forget the sensual pleasures of really perfect tomatoes.

We are at a supermarket at LaSalle and Division in downtown Chicago; Jeff has to circle the parking lot twice before
he finds a spot. The wind blows in bitter and hard off Lake
Michigan a few blocks away; it brings tears to Jeff's lively
eyes, even behind the protection of his glasses, as we stagger
across the icy parking lot, clutching our coats to our chests.

On this bone-rackingly cold day, we are going to buy
tomatoes.

It is midday, and the market is crowded with shoppers.
We head back to the produce department to look at the display of MacGregor tomatoes. Jeff is nominally excited; he
hasn't seen the tomatoes in an actual store yet.

The tomato display features several kinds of tomatoes:
some bleached pink tomatoes that I guess are probably gas-
greened, a supposition with which Jeff agrees; some hydro-

ponic tomatoes, which look and feel like pale red golf balls; the by now ubiquitous pear-shaped Romas, a not-too-bad winter choice since their paste-tomato characteristics guarantee a buyer of at least a reasonable amount of tomato flesh.

There are displayed here, too, some "vine-ripe" beefsteaks; they are priced at $2.99 a pound, and they look unappealingly pink-red. These are tumbled in a bulk bin next to the MacGregor tomatoes, which are priced at $2.59 a pound. Jeff is not pleased with the MacGregor display, which isn't tidily managed and includes tomatoes dumped from their flats into a big, unwieldy pile. "We have to do a lot of in-store education with these guys," he says in the same tone of voice that one might use for a mild curse. "We send the tomatoes perfectly packed in these flats, and look what they do to them."

As we study the tomatoes, a shopper stops to consider a tomato purchase. She looks at the prices: "They're all so expensive!" she says sadly. She looks at the tomatoes themselves; her hand hovers over first the beefsteaks, then the MacGregors, then the Romas. Finally, as if confused by the choices, she turns to Jeff. "Do you know the differences in these tomatoes?" she says. "Well, these are the best," he says, pointing naturally to the MacGregors and slipping a wink to me. "They are? How do you know that?" the woman says, and Jeff answers, "They're my tomatoes."

"You grew them?" she says.

"Well, not exactly," Jeff confesses. "I work for the company that grows them."

"Well, what is the difference, then?" she asks again.

"They're, uh . . . they're, er . . . they're just better, all the way around," stammers Jeff.

"Maybe I'll try them," the woman says, smiling, and makes her selection. Jeff and I choose one tomato, too, and make our way back to the crowded checkout lanes.

At the register, the young cashier inexplicably charges us

the beefsteak tomato price for our MacGregor tomato. Hey, I say pleasantly, that's not the right price. These tomatoes are $2.59 a pound, not $2.99. The cashier looks confused: "The produce manager said to use the same PLU (price look-up) code for the MacGregor tomatoes as for the beefsteak tomatoes," she says, showing us the flip-book price chart as proof. She doesn't know what to do; the line of shoppers behind us is growing longer by the minute. Never mind, I say, and count out the additional change. But I think to myself that this is a shrewd, if dishonest, produce guy: it's a handy forty cents per pound profit for him, an easy-to-miss forty-cent loss for an unwary customer.

On the way to lunch at a hole-in-the-wall eatery that Jeff describes as "the best Mexican restaurant in Chicago," we talk about Calgene's tomato and what its future might be. Jeff, like all the Calgene employees, expects the FDA to approve the tomato in the very near future. He is confident that the buying public will find in this tomato a product worth buying, even at a premium price—a price he says has not yet been set. He tells me that Calgene Fresh has agreed that the public should not subsidize its research by paying an outrageously high price for its tomatoes; I laugh, knowing about the company's expectation of an $8 billion profit in the first year, and say I think that's most generous of the company.

Besides, says Jeff, these tomatoes will be clearly labeled: the buyer will know, if he troubles himself to read the in-store display materials, that these tomatoes are bioengineered. It is right and proper that the public should be allowed to make their own choice about these tomatoes, he says; he thinks that Calgene's tomatoes will have quite a lot of very satisfied buyers.

There is a moment at the airport, when Jeff drops me off, that touches me: I can see him hesitate, torn between an urge to give me a hug and the urge to stay in his professional armor. He settles on the professional, but shakes my hand warmly: we have spent quite a lot of time together in the past few days.

I study him discreetly for the briefest moment. This earnest, well-meaning young man with a hockey stick in the backseat of his Saturn sedan has confessed a secret passion for a life on the land but believes it will not be possible for him. Instead, he has said, he'll try to make some money and maybe be able to buy a vacation house somewhere, a place where he can get away from the stresses of corporate life.

# *3*

# *He Feeds Eighty Families from a Five-Acre Garden*

*K*eeping up with Bruce Schultz's long legs in the knee-deep snow is a challenge for a five-foot-tall person: each of his strides covers a distance nearly two-thirds of my height. He ambles purposefully through the snow; I make my way behind him.

Not that I mind, particularly. We have left the sunny midday warmth of the house to walk the T-shaped parcel of five and a half acres that make up Celebration Gardens, a community-supported agriculture farm that Bruce founded in 1991. It is the most lovely of Michigan winter days, with new snow thick and sparkling on the ground and blue skies overhead. It seems a fine day to be outside, and a fine day, as well, to think about what this small plot of land can accomplish.

Celebration Gardens is in the community of Comstock, eight or ten miles east of Kalamazoo, toward the western side of Michigan. Bruce appreciates with wry wit his efforts to see a sustainable agriculture enterprise blossom in the very shadow of industrial-style agricultural giant Upjohn; the company and its Asgrow seed division have a number of bio-engineered agricultural products awaiting government approval, and Upjohn is a leading manufacturer of herbicides, pesticides, fertilizers, and veterinary medicines. Upjohn's international headquarters lies just a handful of miles away; we could walk there in about an hour.

At forty-four, Bruce is a lean, handsome man with silvered dark hair and a fine hawk's-bill nose. His eyes are merry, and so is his manner: "I'm ready to talk seriously now," he says, slipping a toy toucan beak over his own nose. He and his wife, Christine Kvarnverg, share the responsibilities for household, cooking, and child care about equally it would seem; our conversation on this day will pause several times while Bruce tends to the needs of their daughters, five-year-old Eretia and three-year-old Paige, or their shy one-year-old son, Jacob.

But Bruce is no simpleton, despite his tomfoolery. Born and raised in New York City, Bruce has spent the bulk of his life searching for something exactly like he's found here in Comstock: land to garden on, trees and wildlife, and a way of living that respects the land. It is this vision that led Bruce from New York City to Chicago to Michigan to California to New York State and back to Michigan, but it is a vision not yet entirely achieved. Both Bruce and Christine work as rehabilitation counselors for blind students at a state training facility nearby; he teaches orientation and travel skills, while Christine teaches daily living skills, cooking and the like. These jobs, not the farm, says Bruce, mostly pay the bills; the couple rarely work the same hours, and for a span of time, she worked days and he worked nights.

Yet paying the bills is obviously not topmost in Bruce's priorities. It is Celebration Gardens that drives him and Celebration Gardens' successes that please him most. The gardens are his baby, after a manner of speaking; asked what her role is in Celebration Gardens, Christine smiles pleasantly and says forthrightly if modestly, "I'm the farmer's wife." Her modesty aside, she has naturally lent great assistance in seeing the project launched.

Community-supported agriculture—sometimes called community shared agriculture or CSA—is a relatively new development on the American agricultural scene but one with ancient roots: ideas like it are commonplace in Europe and Japan. Its premise is that a group of people, the "sharers," will join the farmer in bearing the costs and risks of producing food on the farmer's land, sometimes volunteering labor in amounts established before the season begins. In exchange for their preseason payment and their occasional labor, members get a share of the harvest.

The arrangement is of mutual benefit. Sharers are assured of clean, wholesome food grown on local soils, often from heirloom or older varieties of plants or increasingly rare breeds of stock. The grower is assured of a fair and stable income, which protects his ability to remain on the land; the sharers' payments early in the season offset his heaviest expenses at the beginning of the growing season.

But CSAs are not simply just a new way to get cheap vegetables. It can be said that CSA members express their support for a farmer who produces food and they express it financially, with their annual pledges. The vegetables and fruits and other foods they receive are, you might say, a fringe benefit, albeit a good one. CSAs represent a way of thinking about food that is not grounded in a cash economy, a money psychology. They express an understanding that we all, urban and rural dweller alike, depend on the farm to provision us, and they return to the farmer the dignity and respect that agribusiness has stripped from him.

At most CSAs the farmer or gardener retains the responsibility for growing methods, and sharers understand that it is the farmer's job to do this in the best way he or she knows how. And CSA farmers say that, freed from near-constant worries about profit and loss, they can concentrate more completely on the work of growing food.

Celebration Gardens had fifty-five sharers at the outset of the 1993 growing season; some had purchased full shares at about $500, enough fruit and vegetables for a family of two adults and two children or two adult vegetarians through the twenty-week season; others had purchased half shares at $265. Some members paid cash for their share. Some paid a little extra to excuse themselves from the agreement to work a minimum of two hours a month. Others agreed to work more hours in exchange for a chance to spend less money. A few shares, including Bruce's, were all-work, no-cash shares, promising a minimum of a hundred hours' labor over the season. He works in the gardens every day before leaving for the rehabilitation job at four p.m., as do another full-time gardener and two part-timers.

Members include all manner of people: one is a nun, whose order, the Sisters of Saint Joseph, has a retirement home and the order's mother house nearby; others are professional people who want their kids involved in the growing of their food, who want their children to learn more about nature than they could in a one-day workshop.

At the moment Celebration Gardens offers only produce, although Bruce hopes to add more livestock—there are bees here, to help in pollination—sometime in the future; many of the more than three hundred CSAs around the country produce eggs, meat, and milk as well as fruits and vegetables.

Bruce keeps careful, detailed records, so it's easy to track what Celebration Gardens' members got for their investment of faith, work, and money in the '93 garden.

Forty-four crops were planted in Celebration Gardens' various plots, each named for the closest notable tree standing over it. The variety of foodstuffs raised on this small parcel of land is worth detailing; these amounts are totals earned by a whole share. All these foods were raised organically; in fact, the Michigan Department of Agriculture has used both broccoli and carrots from Celebration Gardens as the benchmark controls to monitor chemical residues on produce from other growers.

Each full-share participant in Celebration Gardens' 1993 season received:

Basil, 3.4 pounds
Green and Romano beans, 27.7 pounds
Beets, 16.5 pounds
Broccoli, 7.8 pounds
Cabbage, 9 pounds
Carrots, 18.2 pounds
Cauliflower, .8 pound
Cilantro, .38 pound
Collard greens, 5.5 pounds
Cucumbers, 8.8 pounds
Dill, .45 pound
Eggplant, 9.1 pounds
Flowers, 2.2 pounds
Garlic, 2 pounds
Kale, 3.4 pounds
Leeks, 5 pounds
Lettuce, 18.3 pounds

Melons, 14.2 pounds
Onions, 10.4 pounds
Parsley, 1.5 pounds
Parsnips, .9 pound
Peas, 1.5 pounds
Green peppers, 5.1 pounds
Red peppers, 2.8 pounds
Hot peppers, .6 pound
White and red potatoes, 26.8 pounds
Pie pumpkins, 8.5 pounds
Carving pumpkins, 12.2 pounds
Radishes, 4 pounds
Raspberries, 1 pound
Rhubarb, 2.5 pounds
Scallions, 1.1 pounds
Spinach, 4.3 pounds
Patty pan squash, 11 pounds
Winter squash, 6.7 pounds
Yellow squash, 17.7 pounds
Zucchini, 10.3 pounds
Strawberries, 2.5 pounds
Swiss chard, 5.4 pounds
Cherry tomatoes, 2.78 pounds
Tomatoes, 22.5 pounds
Summer turnips, 3 pounds
Winter turnips, 1 pound

Shareholders could also help themselves to surplus vegetables set aside by other shareholders who happened not to care for that vegetable. They were able to pick, within reason, as much basil, flowers, Swiss chard, raspberries, strawberries, collard greens, kale, hot peppers, and herb garden plants as they wished. Celebration Gardens also donated $676 in food to Ministry with Community, a local food bank.

Over the course of the 20-week growing season, Celebration Gardens produced 21,698 pounds of food. The diversity of crops grown on Celebration Gardens' small acreage is the antithesis of a monocrop enterprise. But that diversity acts in part as insurance against crop failure because of drought, disease, or pest problems. Even if one crop does poorly, others are likely to do well; enough food is produced in the end to feed everyone associated with the farm.

Bruce calculated the retail dollar value of a shareholder's harvest at $332.21 for the 1993 season, those low numbers reflecting some crop failures that summer, but he and the shareholders agree that the money isn't the point. Part of the principle of community-supported agriculture is that members share risks—and bountiful harvests, too—with the farmer.

"People inevitably come to us with a dollars-per-pound attitude," says Bruce. "What we do here is beyond that: we're using this place for our healing and enlightenment, and in the process, the earth is healed, too. Personally, I find a lot of reward in working the earth. To me there's nothing nobler. It's my meditation." Other members agree. Wrote Marcy Clark-Lee in one of the Gardens' newsletters, "The other day I was out harvesting beans in the gardens and began thinking and talking about what picking beans is like for me . . . how a simple daily act (with potential for boredom) turns into a metaphor—a lesson of how to approach life, or maybe an instruction on how I have approached life."

Moreover, says Bruce, the gardens work to heal the community they support and are supported by. "I've been understanding the importance of doing things in your own community and keeping that money at home," he says. "And I also wanted to do my little bit to stop urban sprawl. To have this be a working farm is cool; to have this be an organic farm is even better."

Finally, says Bruce, there is a spiritual aspect to this system of food production that he finds very important. "We have to connect with our God, and this is one way to do it," he says. "By working the earth in this way, we help bring energy to heal the whole community."

Despite those virtues, he says, the Gardens' progress has been fitful. In 1991 when Celebration Gardens began, Bruce hoped for sixty shareholders; when the gardens were planted in the spring, they had 30½ paying shares, 5½ working shares, and enough planted for 40 shares, with the hope that a few more shareholders could be recruited. In the 1992 planning sessions, Bruce held hopes for seventy paid shares and seven working shares; by June that had settled down to 53½ paid shares and 7 working shares. He hoped to reach the seventy-five-member mark in 1993, too, but ended the season with 55; to recover some income from the planned-for-but-not-taken shares, Bruce and other members sold surplus produce at the Kalamazoo farmers market each Saturday, and to local food co-ops and restaurants. That might not have been the best use of their time, Bruce says, but on the other hand, it did give Celebration Gardens an opportunity to reach some potential shareholders who might otherwise have never known about the farm.

Bruce thinks the reason for these struggles is that people don't understand how a community-supported farm works; some don't believe they have the time or energy to provision themselves in this way, and others think the whole proposition is just too much trouble. Those who have signed on have been so happy that they've all returned year after year, except for the members who moved away or were inspired to begin their own gardens. Some would-be shareholders may be daunted by the requirement to pay for their produce in the spring, before they get it, but social justice issues seem important to Bruce, as they are to most CSA farmers I've spoken with: no one has been or would be turned away if he or she couldn't come up with the money to pay for a share. Bruce feels strongly that clean, wholesome food is a natural human right, and as is typical of most CSAs, Celebration Gardens makes every effort to accommodate the special needs of people with lower incomes.

Every possible effort, that is. "Food stamps are a sad story," says Bruce. "I applied to the Grand Rapids regional office of the United States Department of Agriculture (which administers the food stamps program)—and they rejected me. I appealed that decision and was rejected again. I heard that a CSA near Ann Arbor was able to arrange that for its shareholders (through a different regional office), but I couldn't do it—they said because people were paying first and getting food later, and because there wasn't a strict dollars-for-product exchange." So Celebration Gardens' lower-income shareholders may pay in installments or work extra hours in exchange for a lower cash investment in their share, or "volunteer" for an all-work, no-cash share, if any are available.

Celebration Gardens shareholders have struggled with another problem, says Bruce. Its members who have become used to choosing only broccoli-carrots-tossed salads often don't know how to prepare vegetables like kale and collard greens, bok choy and parsnips. Sometimes they want to learn: the quarterly newsletter that Celebration Gardens publishes often features recipes from its members. But sometimes members don't know or aren't interested in learning, and those vegetables are underused. They may end up on the surplus table, from which unclaimed produce goes to local food banks and feeding programs. Bruce feels, and I agree, that some of the Gardens' members are missing an opportunity to broaden their palates and their horizons.

Shareholders also don't know how to can or preserve their own gardens' surplus, says Bruce, and they usually don't want to know. He mentions that he was offered a complete commercial canning kitchen for the cost of dismantling it and taking it away, but the members weren't enthusiastic about the idea and so the offer went unaccepted. This surprises me, as it does him, but we agree that it must be a combination of not knowing how to preserve food and thinking the work is too much trouble to be worth the investment of time. Still, the idea of seeing food you've helped raise go to waste is an odd one to me; it is simply unfathomable to someone who assigns a high value to food.

But food isn't always the premier reason why Celebration Gardens' shareholders sign on. Members cite a variety of reasons for joining: to support the local economy; to "have their hands in the dirt," as Bruce puts it; and to fit in or find a place in the community. "The gardens replace church for some of our members," says Bruce.

The Gardens' quarterly newsletter announces in nearly every issue an upcoming festival or potluck for its members: a lot of effort is put into creating a sense of community for and among the members. Bruce and Christine open their own home to members—"We tell them they should walk right in, that there's no need to knock, but they aren't always comfortable with that," says Bruce—and make the in-ground swimming pool available to all the Gardens' members. I say that I don't think I could be quite that welcoming, since my needs for privacy would perhaps conflict with such an open-door approach. Bruce laughs and says, "We love living in the village hall! The kids think all these people are coming to visit them, and we're glad to have the company."

Bruce stops in the garden now to pick some stiffly frozen kale, still green and not only edible but improved by its natural icing down. "It's just about done for the year," he says, laying the big leaves in a plastic milk crate for easier handling. He hefts the milk crate easily to his shoulder and ambles back to the house.

Back in the dining room, the still-frozen kale stacked in its crate in the shed outside the kitchen door, Bruce shakes off the winter cold and rubs his stockinged feet to warm them up again.

He believes that the Kalamazoo area could support "a thousand, two thousand" CSAs, and he hopes to see that happen someday. "I want Celebration Gardens to be a prototype; I want people to see that this is fun," he says. But it will take a while.

To my surprise he is undismayed by Celebration Gardens' struggles. Instead, he says philosophically, "You can't push a river. We went into this backwards, trying to organize it from the farm, rather than the other way around. I've been turning more control over to the members, encouraging them to be responsible for more of the decisions. That's the only way this can work."

And this small plot of land may not be where Bruce and his family remain forever in any case. "We need a place with some water—a lake or a stream," he says. That would make livestock possible, an idea that Bruce heartily supports but one that he does not feel comfortable pursuing at the moment.

There are other struggles for Bruce and Christine. One is learning to think about their work at Celebration Gardens as work on a farm, even though it's such a small piece of land. "That's been a major struggle for me," confesses Christine. "It's been hard for me to think of this as a real farm because 'real' farms are bigger."

But Bruce's eyes light up as he thinks about spring and the hurry of labor that begins when the ground thaws and the land is able to be worked at last after a long winter. "We'll be having our spring meeting soon," he says, "and then we can get to work again. That's when the fun begins; that's the exciting time."

The shadows lie long on the snow as we prepare to leave

in the late afternoon. Yet another snowstorm is predicted for today, and the clouds piling up to the west bespeak a truthfulness in the prediction. Soon Bruce will have to leave for the rehabilitation center, and he needs some time to get ready for that work.

He isn't rushing us on our way, however. Instead, he encourages us to come again, to come anytime, to come sometime when the gardens are flourishing and the members are out in full force. Stop by, he says, whenever you find yourself on this side of the state. Come and talk to the members, visit for as long as you like.

Everyone is welcome at Celebration Gardens.

## THE HISTORY OF CSA

The CSA movement in this country may be said to have begun at Indian Line Farm in Great Barrington, Massachusetts, in 1985. A hundred years ago the rich soil of the Berkshires was home to innumerable farmers; but now few farmers work the land there.

Back in 1985 a group of Great Barrington residents came together to form what they called the CSA Garden; the group sold thirty shares in an apple orchard, with share costs determined by the expenses of picking, sorting, storing, and distributing 360 bushels of apples.[1] Some of the apples were pressed for cider, hard cider, and vinegar, and all the products were shared among the members. The success of the project convinced the members that the idea of a community-supported agricultural enterprise could work.

At the same time, members of the group arranged to rent some land from Robyn Van En of Indian Line Farm in South

---

[1] For more on CSAs in America, see *Farms of Tomorrow: Community Supported Farms, Farm Supported Communities* by Trauger M. Groh and Steven S. H. McFadden (Biodynamic Farming and Gardening Association, Kimberton, PA, 1990).

Egremont, Massachusetts; Robyn was a member of the garden's core group, the handful of people who worked especially hard to see the project succeed. The three-year lease included an option to buy and also made available water, electricity, vehicle access, and the use of an outbuilding. As the apples neared the end of their harvest, the members plowed, composted, manured, harrowed, and planted cover crops so the rented acres would be ready for cultivation in the spring.

The core group met during the months that the land slept, planning and hammering out the details of the garden they would plant. They estimated that a share should include four to six hundred pounds of vegetables per year and planned their production accordingly. They decided to plant forty to fifty different kinds of vegetables, herbs, flowers, and mushrooms.

By spring planting some fifty shares had been sold, enough to get the garden off the ground. By 1989 its membership had grown to some 150 shares, which was about as much as the land could support, and the Great Barrington CSA split into two CSAs, Indian Line Farm and Sunways Farm.

From the earliest days the Great Barrington CSA set out to include all the members of its community. Mentally handicapped residents from Berkshire Village took part, both as growers and as members. John Root, Jr., another core-group Great Barrington CSA member, argued that the need for a decent, dignified life is in all of us, whatever our skills, and the rest of the members agreed.

CSAs offer strong economic benefits for local economies, since less money flows from a community to more distant points.

"Massachusetts imports approximately 85 to 90 percent of its food," says Robyn, who helped found the Great Barrington CSA and still lives on Indian Line Farm. "That means almost $4 billion a year leaks out of the state's economy—and the figures are consistent with almost every other state in the union. But Massachusetts could be producing closer to 35 percent of its own food, which would keep nearly $1 billion in the Commonwealth. Depending upon how innovative and resourceful our agriculture strategies are, it could possibly be more."

She also speaks of a level of economic insurance for the farmer, possible with CSAs but impossible under conventional market-driven systems.

"During the first CSA year at Indian Line Farm, a freak thunderstorm dropped eight inches of rain in three hours," she says. "Due to the integrated cropping and disc-harrow raised beds, the winter storage squash was the only real loss. It was harvested in premature condition, and members cooked or froze whatever they wanted. This translated to a $35 loss on each share purchase—but would have been a $3500 loss to the farm family on a conventional farm."

Trauger Groh, who coauthored *Farms of Tomorrow*, helped start the Great Barrington CSA with advice and counsel he had gained while studying CSAs in Europe, although he settled on another CSA in New Hampshire. "The problems of agriculture and the environment belong not just to a small minority of active farmers," Trauger writes in *Farms of Tomorrow*, "they are the problems of all humanity."

He argues eloquently that foods from an integrated, balanced local farm will provide higher-quality nutrition and will improve soil, water, air quality, and other environmental values.

But he also argues that there are many important lessons for all of us to learn from the farm, lessons we have forgotten or never learned since we left the farm behind.

I think of my own childhood, when I used to visit a friend whose family owned a dairy farm. In the summer we

sometimes worked with her brother or father, "tucking
string." It was the local name for the hot, dirty, scratchy
work of walking along behind a hay baler and snugging the
twine that held the rectangular bales together. As we got
older the job included loading the bales onto a flatbed wagon,
and my friend taught me a trick. The bales are heavy, so you
pick them up only high enough to bounce them off your
thighs and onto the wagon. That was why we didn't wear
cutoffs while baling hay: the bales would have chafed our legs
into bloodied soreness if we had. By tucking string I learned
that there is usually a trick to doing a job right—but that the
job must be done, however unpleasant it might be.

Best of all, perhaps, I learned that even an unpleasant
job comes to an end.

In visiting that farm I learned other things, too. No matter how small or young we were, there was work for us to do,
and doing it well made us feel proud because even the small
work was important. Seeing that the calves were fed was as
necessary as getting the cows milked. We saw that careless-
ness was no excuse for doing a thing improperly; a gate left
unhitched could mean the ruin of a field of corn.

I learned a lot about living on my visits to that farm, but
not all of it was work. I discovered how sweet a loft full of hay
smells, and that if you chew on fresh wheat for a little while,
it turns into what my friend called "farmer's gum." I tasted
milk fresh from the cow, still warm from her body, and found
that chickens won't hurt you when you take away their eggs
if you are fast and sure-handed. I saw the fields when they
were raw and bare in the spring, and full and fecund in
the fall.

Trauger Groh writes that three motivations must come
together for these community-supported agriculture farms—
the "farms of tomorrow"—to succeed. The first is spiritual,
that life may be created fresh each year on the land, and that

human beings may be born into and nurture healthy bodies. The second is social: to shape land so everyone has the healthful food, wood, and fiber he needs. The final motivation is economic: the ideal is a farm that is economically sound, maintaining high fertility through careful management, fertility that rewards its community with a surplus of food.

I cannot help but wonder when the last time an agribusiness company concerned itself with spiritual and social mores, when such a company considered any economic survival beyond its own. It is, after all, not the business of business to look after such esoteric ideals; it is the business of business to make money.

## GROWING GARDENERS AND GARDENS

Will Raap is the kind of man who radiates a peaceful yet purposeful energy. His company, Gardener's Supply of Burlington, Vermont, has been successful in the competitive gardening industry, selling by mail-order and retail outlet tools, seeds, and garden extras. And while Will works as hard as anyone who works for him—the day I visit, he has spent a couple of hours on the mail-order phone lines, as do almost all the employees—he has broadened his search for a new challenge.

He has found it in the Intervale, a 750-acre lowlands in the heart of Burlington, land that was used as late as the 1960s for farming. The Intervale has been farmed since mankind first settled the area, says Will; artifacts of Native American cultures found on the land prove that. "Intervale" is an old word, springing from an agrarian view of land and its worth: the word means bottomland, or land along a river, and as any farmer will tell you, bottomlands are often the most fertile around.

The tall, blond, blue-eyed Will laughs when he explains that his interest in growing things may be genetic: "Raap means 'turnip' in Dutch," he says, grinning. But growing his gardening company wasn't challenging enough, so in 1988 Will and others launched a CSA on twenty acres leased from the city of Burlington in the Intervale, and the successful enterprise is now run by the nonprofit Intervale Foundation. Nearly a hundred families held shares in 1993, says Will, either a group share (enough for four adults: $325 and twelve hours' work in the gardens during the summer) or an individual share (enough for one to two adults: $200 and six hours of work over the summer). The CSA also offers shares for eggs and chicken, and winter shares—filled from stored vegetables and those grown in greenhouses—are available separately for $125 and eight hours' labor.

As is true at Bruce Schultz's CSA, however, members also enjoy festivals and other events that further their sense of connection and community. A harvest festival in September 1993 also celebrated the tenth anniversary of Gardener's Supply, and Will himself led an 8.5-mile bike ride—some of it along new paths and bridges built by Gardener's Supply employees—to open the festival. The bike paths built for the festival were Gardener's Supply's gift to the public. It was, one senses, the kind of day that Will himself enjoys most, surrounded by people who may discover for the first time the pleasures of the land.

Will's business background has given him an appreciation of spreadsheets and the data they can convey. It is in looking at these spreadsheets that the Intervale Foundation's value becomes most evident. Eighteen full- and part-time jobs have been created; the CSA produced $45,000 worth of food in 1993. Other Foundation projects—including cooperative farms, the Vermont Pure Water fish farm, and the Burlington Flower Farm—brought the total value of food produced on the once-abandoned Intervale up to $166,000. Will expects to see that grow to $830,000 by 1995, with a concurrent doubling of jobs created.

But two of the Foundation's projects warrant special attention.

The Intervale Foundation has arranged with the city of Burlington to compost both yard wastes and food scraps produced by city residents. The compost enriches the land in the Intervale at a rate of more than four thousand tons of compost in 1993 alone. At a landfill dumping fee of $74 a ton, Will figures the composting program saved the city nearly $312,000, no small shakes for a small city's budget, and no small shakes, either, to the landfill spared that additional burden.

Additional food waste for composting comes from the Medical Center Hospital of Vermont, a stone's throw away from the Intervale. In 1993 the hospital's director of nutrition services, Michael Kanfer, agreed to buy some twenty thousand pounds of vegetables grown in a special Foundation-run one-acre market garden in the Intervale. Kanfer committed $20,000 to $30,000 of his $150,000 annual fresh produce budget to the project, and hopes he'll be able to buy eighty thousand pounds of produce in the future.

The produce is grown organically, as are all the fruits and vegetables in the Intervale Foundation's gardens. And judging by Kanfer's remarks in a September 1993 issue of *FoodService Director*, the project has been a ripping success. "Our people are absolutely amazed at the quality—it's no more than four hours from the garden to the kitchen," Kanfer said.

His staff met with gardeners at the Foundation, who agreed to grow kale, lettuce, tomatoes, green peppers, carrots, strawberries, and several other foods possible in Vermont's short growing season. The hospital agreed to pay a premium of twenty percent over the price it would have paid a distributor for the same amount of food, a premium for its organic cultivation and its very high quality.

The hospital also agreed to truck about a ton of food waste each week back to the Intervale Foundation for composting, for which it pays the Foundation $50 a ton—still less than the $74 a ton the hospital used to pay to have the waste hauled away and dumped into the landfill.

It seems to be a win-win-win situation, says Will: patients at the hospital get the freshest locally grown organic produce possible; local farmers have a market for their products; and the Foundation—and the land—benefit from the composted food scraps.

Will says the Foundation hopes to attract other commercial and institutional members—local restaurants, schools, anyone who buys and prepares food for the public. He is sure, given the successes already achieved in the Foundation's five-year life, that these ideas are not only feasible but profitable for all involved.

Darkness has fallen as I prepare to leave the Intervale with Will at the end of the day. I realize, as I hike along Burlington's quiet evening streets, that I feel more optimistic about the possibility of change than I have ever felt before. What Will has wrought in Burlington works, and it can work anywhere. This I lay at Will's feet: several of his employees had told me earlier in the day that he has this effect on people.

## *HOW FAR ARE YOU FROM YOUR SUPPER?*

There is a penciled note, addressed to me by name, taped to Brewster Kneen's door when I arrive at his Toronto home. "I will be right back," it says. "Please wait." I am happy to do so: despite a lowering sky of overcast pewter, the day is pleasant, and Brewster's stoop is broad and inviting. I plop down and study the little garden to one side of the front yard; it is perhaps ten feet by five, and the tall stakes tell me that the withered husks entwined about them were once bean and tomato plants.

Fewer than ten minutes pass before Brewster rides up on a bicycle, his pant legs bound by clips. There is a small, older economy car in the driveway, but he tells me, as we go into the house, that he and his wife, Cathleen, rarely use it.

Brewster is a silver-haired, lean fellow in his early sixties; he and Cathleen edit a monthly newsletter on agricultural issues and food system analysis called *The Ram's Horn*, and Brewster is the author of *From Land to Mouth: Understanding the Food System* (NC Press, 1989; 1993). Brewster emigrated to Canada in 1965, where he became a peace activist. He has also worked as a radio broadcaster, a social justice organizer, and corporate critic. He speaks and writes often of his own and his wife's Christian faith.

Brewster points to a framed photo of a cornfield that hangs on one living room wall: "There," he says, "is the secret to why agriculture isn't working anymore." The cornfield looks lush, the plants themselves look green and healthy. The ground between the rows is bare, giving the field a well-groomed look. "That's the way a lot of people think a cornfield should look," says Brewster. "But the only way to keep that ground bare between the rows is to spray herbicides to keep down the weeds. A lot of herbicides."

It is Brewster's contention that we began to distance ourselves from food quite naturally, as an outgrowth of economic and social thinking that began in seventeenth- and eighteenth-century England. As we turned from a society founded on religious and agrarian principles to one founded on scientific thinking, he says, we began the natural commodification of food. We stopped thinking of food as something that was grown, and began to think of it as something that had to be produced, like steel or manufactured goods.

Yet Brewster recalls the 15 years he and Cathleen lived on a Nova Scotia farm. "We grew forage crops and raised beef cattle, sheep, chickens, dogs, and two children," he says. "We regarded ourselves as farmers. We never thought of referring to ourselves as 'children producers.' " During that period, however, he and Cathleen would have been properly described, in our current way of thinking about agriculture, as "beef producers," as "sheep producers," as "poultry producers."

In other words, says Brewster, when farmers stop thinking of themselves as farmers, whose principal work is the growing of food, and start thinking of themselves as businessmen, whose chief aim is to make a profit, the system begins to distance us from our food supply.

Distancing works in many ways, on many levels, he says. There is more distance between the place where the food is grown and the place where it is eaten than there was a hundred years ago; there is more distance between the time the food is harvested and the time it is eaten; and there is especially more distance between the farmer and the people he feeds—psychologically, philosophically, economically, and physically.

The antidote to distancing is, quite logically, proximity. "Food should be consumed as close to the point and condition of production as possible," says Brewster. "Another way of describing proximity is to say that the closer the food source is to the consumer, the less money is required for nutrition. An economic system that seeks to maximize the amount of money that can be made out of anything will pursue the logic of distancing, not proximity."

Brewster Kneen thinks a lot about food and its commodification. He thinks a lot, too, about the idea that anyone should be forced to pay for food, the idea that wholesome, clean food and enough of it isn't a natural human right. He couches these thoughts in the metaphor of his deep Presbyterian faith. "To insist that nourishment—salvation—must be purchased is immoral and sinful," he says. And he strengthens his point by quoting from Isaiah 55:1: "Oh, come to the water, all you who are thirsty; though you have no money, come! Buy corn without money, and eat, and, at no cost, wine and milk."

# The Business of Dairying Today

*W*hen Ken Nobis of Saint Johns, Michigan, tells you he won a full football scholarship for the last three years of college, it comes as no surprise. Nobis is big, broad through the shoulders, and sturdy; his deep-set ice blue eyes sometimes shine with merriment, but are usually stern beneath his sandy brows. At fifty, Nobis needs glasses for reading, but when he walks the barns and lanes of the farm, he leaves the glasses off. His shaggy hair, graying only slightly, pops out from under the "gimme" cap—baseball caps given as promotional items by agricultural concerns—he wears indoors and out.

Nobis and his brother, Larry, are partners in Nobis Dairy Farms; Larry oversees the crop production—crops that will feed the cattle—while Ken looks after dairy affairs. Together they are the third generation on this farm, founded by their grandfather in the mid 1940s. The farm has grown, shrunk, and shifted in ownership through the generations, but today the Nobis brothers survey some six hundred acres and 550 holsteins and call it their own. The land is mostly flat with only gentle rises; woodlots dot the landscape occasionally, but most of the fields are planted virtually to the road's edge. On the home farm, where Ken and Larry grew up, most of the old barns and sheds are gone, replaced by newer metal pole-barn buildings.

The Nobis brothers were among the first farmers in the country to experiment with a controversial bioengineered hormone injected in cows to make them give more milk. The hormone, called recombinant bovine somatotropin (rBST) by its supporters and recombinant bovine growth hormone (rBGH) by its critics, mimics a hormone that cows produce naturally. To distinguish between the natural and bioengineered varieties, I'll refer to the synthetic version as rBST/rBGH. We'll talk more later about the drug and the Nobises' experiences with it while they tested the drug in its preapproval stages for the Monsanto Company, the first company to win FDA approval for the hormone.

Ken says his family's roots were in Illinois; his grandfather, Walter, came to Michigan from there in the "nineteen-teens," he says. Walter worked as a sharecropper until the middle of World War II, when he purchased this farm and formed a partnership with his three sons; in that period, the farm's holdings expanded. Although the partnership dissolved in the '60s, Ken and Larry have rebuilt their holdings, nearly matching the seven hundred acres their grandfather, father, and uncles held.

"I grew up dairying, but I didn't have it in mind to farm," remembers Ken, as he sits in the office built where the family's chicken coop used to be. Two computers occupy

Ken's desk; when he works at them, he looks at either a blank wall with only a calendar on its dark paneling or at a wall festooned with more than a dozen state dairying and soil conservation awards. The changing computer screen of one advertises the availability of up-to-the-minute market prices from the Chicago exchanges; the other is dedicated to herd and farm records, it would seem. An official-looking portrait of the Nobises' father hangs on the wall by the awards: he looks prosperous, serious, and intent. By contrast, Larry's desk overlooks an open barn—where heifers are kept until they are bred—and the fields beyond.

Ken Nobis went to Western Michigan University, thinking he'd do two years there before transferring to Michigan State University, the state's premier agriculture school. But when he won that full football scholarship in his second year, he decided to stay at Western. He majored in agriculture, graduating in 1966.

That timing is important: the young Ken came home after graduation and worked for his father on the farm for just two months before being drafted. Looking back, he says he "didn't mind" going into the army. And indeed it could be said that Ken was a lucky Vietnam-era soldier: he spent twenty months stationed in Germany, where he worked as a clerk. He was the first of his college friends to be drafted, and one of only two who were drafted who didn't go to Vietnam.

Like many of his peers in that era, the farmer's son married a girl he met at college—Liz Mejers—rather than the daughter of a neighboring farmer. He and his wife have raised two sons, Kerry, twenty-four, who lives at home and works on the farm; and Mitch, twenty-one, who's studying at the University of Michigan to be a teacher. There are no photos of his family on Ken's desk, and we do not meet Liz today; she works off the farm.

Neither Nobis family lives on the farm anymore; the two

white frame houses are made available to employees as perks, as are the sides of beef from the few beef cattle raised on the farm. Both Nobises have built newer houses on land close by.

In fact, says Ken, he doesn't even drink milk from his own cows: he prefers to buy it, pasteurized and homogenized, at the grocery store in town. This is in part because a bout of bovine brucellosis on the farm when he was a teen meant the milk had to be dumped, and since then he's grown to prefer the store-bought stuff. But it is also true that for Ken milk is "product," and product is meant for sale.

"If I hadn't been drafted, I would have gone into industry," says Ken. "I would have accepted one of the half-dozen job offers I had then, probably would have taken an offer from International Harvester as an industrial management trainee."

But the job offer was long gone when Ken came home from the army, so he and his young family settled in at the farm. "In May of 1971 I formed a partnership with my dad," he says. "Larry was working for a feed company in upstate New York then; he came back and joined the partnership in 1974."

The early '70s marked a period of new expansion in the Nobis family's farm holdings. They bought a neighbor's farm in 1973, bringing the farm up to its current nearly six hundred acres. In 1968 father and son milked about sixty-five cows; by 1974 that had nearly doubled. By 1994 the partnership milked 550 holsteins, about twenty percent purebred registered cows and the balance unregistered cows. Asking a farmer the value of his cows is a form of rural rudeness; it's as nosy as asking to peek in his wallet. But nationally, depending on their bloodlines, holsteins range in value from $2,500 to $10,000 or more. It's a safe bet that most of Ken's cows are valued from the mid to high end of that range.

Perhaps more remarkable, however, is the change in the "rolling herd average" for milk production at Nobis Farms since Ken returned from the army. A rolling herd average is the farm's total yearly milk production divided by the number of cows on the farm. It is a good measure of productivity because it is a standard measurement even when the number of cows rises or falls. When Ken returned from the army, the farm's rolling herd average was about twelve thousand pounds of milk per cow. Today, some twenty-five years later, it's just about double that.

There are three keys to that rise in production, Ken says. "Some of it's genetics, some of it's environmental, and some of it's nutrition—and not necessarily in that order. We've become a lot more conscious about the stresses in a cow that lower milk production, and we've learned a great deal about how cow nutrition can improve production."

The Nobises have always been early adopters of technology; they've always looked for new ways and styles of doing things, always with the idea of improving their rolling herd average. As an example, the Nobises had the second loafing shed in Clinton County; they built it in 1956, after a tornado blew down one of the farm's barns. Loafing sheds, open on the sides to the elements in good weather but usually equipped with adjustable plastic tarps that can close them in bad weather, have come to be the barn of choice among most dairy farmers; farmers have learned that even in the bitter winters of the upper Midwest, it isn't the cold that threatens their cattle, it's the icy winds. In fact, cows suffer worse in summer's high humidity and temperatures than they do in winter. Barns don't need to be heated, but they do need to be well ventilated in both summer and winter.

The Nobis cows have not been on open pasture since loafing sheds were introduced on the farm. From their birth to the day they are culled from the herd, the cows spend their days penned in the barns. It is easier for the farmer, this style of herd management. Chances are you will never again see Nobis cows grazing at peace in open fields.

Ken says, too, that the farm's dairy production took a big leap upward when they adopted the practice of segregating the youngest cows from the older ones, an idea they picked up from dairy scientists at Michigan State University. The young cows aren't assertive enough to push in for their share of food and water, he says, and by keeping the cows in groups of about the same age, the competition—a milk-inhibiting stress—is reduced. So all the cows at Nobis Farms are housed in a series of barns depending on their ages.

We start out from the office to tour the farm on a blustery, sunny midspring day. The tour will start in the maternity area, where cows nearing the end of their pregnancy are housed. As we walk through the airy open barn, we see that one cow in an open stall with a half-dozen others is already well advanced in labor; her sides heave and she groans as she works to deliver her calf. Look, I say, you're about to have another calf. Ken studies the cow with a quick, practiced eye and says he'll have to find someone to move her to a different stall, where she can give birth in peace. I do not routinely watch cows give birth and so wished we could have lingered, but Ken has seen this event thousands of times in his life. One of the ten full-time employees—whom Ken refers to as "full-time equivalents"—will tend to the cow, and he will continue to give the tour and me his attentions.

He points out the recycled newspaper, shredded and spread to a depth of several inches, in a different part of the same barn. Here cows in various stages of pregnancy are housed; a few hours before they deliver, they will be moved into the barn we just walked through. The newspapers are dry and rustling on this fine spring day; Ken says they need only be changed when they've been sodden with urine or rain, but when the warming dry winds of spring blow, it may be several days between changes. The air in this and the rest of the barns is clean and even sweet if the natural odors of cows and their wastes do not offend you. There certainly is no unpleasant ammonia smell, the sign of bad housekeeping on a dairy farm.

From this barn we backtrack a little to the enclosure that Larry Nobis sees when he sits at his desk. Here, newly bred heifers—young cows being bred to their first pregnancy—are settled in. Most of the breeding on Nobis Farms is done by artificial insemination (AI), says Ken, an improvement that makes better bloodlines possible without the hazard and cost of keeping a bull. It became the standard for dairymen in the '60s and '70s. But a younger bull is kept in with these heifers, to "catch" any cows that didn't become pregnant with AI. The heifers are curious, and as Ken leans on the wood gate, they draw near him; he rubs one absently on the neck as he says that when the young bulls start to get "too ornery," he gets rid of them—usually selling them to slaughter.

It is a natural fact that a cow gives milk only after she's borne a calf, so dairy cattle are bred every year while they are productive. A cow may be productive for as few as three years or for many more; cows that no longer earn their keep are culled from the herd and sold at livestock auctions. Most of these animals are destined for the slaughterhouse: McDonald's is the largest purchaser of dairy cow beef in the world.

The Nobises keep every female calf their cows deliver; these calves are needed as eventual replacements for their dams and grandams. The bull calves are culled early from the herd; these, too, are sold at livestock auction as "bob veal," calves that will be raised in various ways, some humane, some less so, for their delicately flavored meat. The heifer calves will stay with their mothers for a few days, since the first few days' milk, called colostrum, provides the calves with natural disease resistance and gives them good nutrition.

Besides, the milk from a cow that has just given birth can't be sold for at least three days. Soon afterward, however, the calves are separated from their dams and moved to a separate area a few hundred yards away. The calves are fed with powdered milk replacer—cheaper than sacrificing the milk the mother produces—and eventually weaned onto dry feeds. It will be more than a year before these heifer calves will be bred for the first time.

Meanwhile, the calves' mothers have rejoined the milking herd. Twice each day they'll make their way into the milking parlor, where machines are attached to their udders and the milk is pumped directly through stainless-steel lines to the holding tank. There it will be quickly cooled to just under forty degrees, and the milk will be held until the milk hauler comes to pick it up. Nobis Farms' cows produce so much milk that it's worth the independent milk hauler's while to pick up every day; at smaller farms the truck may pick up only every other day.

The Nobises used to milk three times a day—they did while they were testing rBST/rBGH for Monsanto—but Ken says now that it's unlikely they'll return to that pattern. Moving more than five hundred cows twice a day is a headache; doing so three times a day is logistically hectic, and it requires more employees to milk three times a day.

But even twice-a-day milking takes a long time. Such a long time, in fact, that the three full-time employees whose job it is solely to milk during the week will begin milking around six a.m. and continue almost all day long, until evening milking is finished around eleven-thirty or midnight. The employees work overlapping shifts, says Ken; the first comes in around two a.m. and begins by cleaning every piece of equipment carefully. Some of the cleaning process is automated; hot water, detergent, and disinfectant are pumped through the lines automatically, and the milk tank cleans itself in the same way. But the milking parlor must be hosed down, and various other parts of the equipment must be washed by hand. Since the milking parlor is open to the south, where the cows come into the parlor, one can imagine that it must be a bitter, cold job on a hard winter's night to do this cleaning.

The first employee finishes his shift at around ten a.m., and by then the second milker has come on to see the morning milking to its conclusion. Next, it's time to wash everything again, and the milking parlor will be newly clean when the second employee finishes up in the late afternoon, in time for the last employee to come in for evening milking. It will be well nigh midnight by the time the third milker is finished, and the cycle will begin again in just a few hours.

On weekends two milkers work longer shifts. But one employee can easily handle the 18 cows milking at any given time in the double-herringbone parlor. The cows walk in and settle themselves into slanted stalls, and the worker fits the milking machines to their udders from the sunken work space that allows him to work at shoulder height. He needn't bend over, as farmers traditionally had to do, to reach the cows' udders.

Other things have changed about milking time, too. Farmers used to grain their cows at milking to supplement their rations of hay and other foods. The Nobises no longer do this, since they have devised ways to be sure the cows are getting proper nutrition while they're in the barns. Ken says he thinks the cows are happier this way—with their heads up, they can look around at their neighbors—and it eases both the workload and the amount of unwholesome jostling that the cows get into when there's grain to be had.

A modern cow needs a lot of food every day to keep up her high milk output, and proper nutrition is a big part of keeping that production high. Ken looks at his herd records to give us the average daily figures for a midrange producer on his farm: each day, she'll need 23.5 pounds of high-moisture corn, 3 pounds of wheat middlings (a part of the kernel), 2 pounds of soy hulls (the covering of soybean seeds, not the pods), 3 pounds of mixed vitamins and minerals in a soy meal carrier, 7.5 pounds of soy meal, 5 pounds of fuzzy cotton seeds (a by-product of southern cotton farming that gives the cows both energy and fiber), 10.5 pounds of alfalfa silage, 25 pounds of corn silage, and 11.5 pounds of sudex silage. Sudex is a recent hybrid of sorghum and Sudan grass; silage is the whole plant, chopped up, and it takes the place of hay in the cow's diet. That's more than 90 pounds of food each day, every day, for a midrange-producing cow.

The Nobises don't grow all the feed their cows need—they must buy about a quarter of it, says Ken. They could perhaps grow more, but they follow a careful crop rotation to protect their soil, and in any case, cotton isn't a northern crop. But a special piece of equipment blends the feed in proper proportion so that every mouthful a cow fetches up from the troughs has the proper mix of nutrients for best milk production. Ken is clearly proud of this development, and it's easy to understand why: the haphazard methods of yore didn't get maximum production from every cow. When he plucks up a handful to show me from a feed trough, it is dry and crumbly, multitextured. The cows like it well enough, it appears.

Stocks of the various foodstuffs needed for the blend are stored at several sites near the newly bred heifers' barn. Silage, which used to be stored in silos on the dairy farms I remember from childhood, is today often stored in tightly packed mounds on concrete pads. Little front-loading tractors scoop out the foodstuffs as needed to carry them to the blending machine. Ken flags down an employee driving one of these little tractors to tell him about the cow giving birth in the maternity shed; a few minutes later we can hear him prodding the cow to move. "Hey-yah," he says, "get on out of there! Get up! Get up!" The cow groans in response; I cannot imagine that getting up and walking is something she has a great deal of interest in at the moment.

In another barn Ken points out the concrete floor sloped to a slight degree, which keeps urine and spilled water flowing away from the cows' feet. The concrete is scored, both to give the cows a better footing and to further encourage drainage into the first of several manure lagoons dug, he says, at great expense. The underground lines that carry the sludge from the pits directly to the fields—where it serves as fertilizer for the crops growing to feed the cows—were expensive, too. Some farmers complained of their cows' foot and leg problems when they moved from pasture to concrete, but the Nobises have had the reverse experience: their cows have fewer problems on concrete than they ever had on open pasture.

The cows in this barn are soon to be in season, ready to breed; an employee stands in the broad center aisle of the barn, just watching, to catch the cows in heat as early as possible. He uses a kindling-sized piece of chalk to mark the rumps of cows he suspects are ready to breed; one of the signs is that other cows will mount a cow ready to breed and the chalk mark will be rubbed off. I say that it seems a funny job, to stand and watch cows all day; Ken says it's one of the hardest jobs on the farm to teach and is a special art in the science of modern dairying. A man who can pick out a cow ready to breed is a valuable employee.

As we watch, one of the cows mounts another and, halfway up, slips and falls. It is a tense moment: one of her rear legs shoots out behind her, a particularly dangerous position for a dairy cow, threatening both her leg and her delicate udder. Ken and I are both silent while we wait to see the cow regain her feet. He is relieved, I know, although he says nothing; when I ask him about it, he says that it's a very real possibility that a cow going down like that won't get up again. He unconsciously signals his relief by lifting his cap with his right hand, wiping his forehead with his left hand, and resettling the cap in one fluid motion, a motion he must repeat dozens of times each day.

As we walk from this barn to visit the newly weaned calves, bawling in frustration for their missing milk, we meet Ken's son Kerry. "I'm going on lunch break," the son says to his impassive father after I've been introduced and greeted. "I'll finish mowing when I come back." Kerry is as tall as his father and as broad; he, too, is handsome in a blunt-featured, wholesome way, but the long ponytail streaming down his back hints of some differences in style from his contained, composed father. Ken says his son hasn't made up his mind about farming yet, says he's still searching for his calling.

Later, Ken tells me that he is very firm with the employees: they must take breaks as the law requires, even if they don't want to. Many of them don't like that, he says, and I say that I can understand their thinking: one gets caught up in one's work if the work is likable. But they have to take breaks, says Ken; I ask why. Because their productivity drops, he explains; the records and study after study prove it. I realize that in meeting various employees, I have seen a great deal of respect for Ken; I have not, however, seen any jocularity, any good-natured teasing or badinage. This is business, after all.

## FROM LAB TO FARM LANE

When the St. Louis–based chemical giant Monsanto needed farmers to conduct field trials of its version of rBGH/rBST, it consulted dairy marketing cooperatives in a number of states. Monsanto is one of four companies that have worked to develop versions of the bioengineered hormone. Upjohn, American Cyanamid, and Eli Lilly have not pressed the FDA for approval of their versions, perhaps preferring to see how Monsanto fares with Posilac, its brand name for rBGH/rBST.

A new veterinary drug has to clear a number of FDA hurdles as it is developed. One of the earliest is the human safety test—would the meat or milk from animals treated with this drug be safe for human consumption? Monsanto provided data to the FDA that convinced scientists there in 1985 that yes, indeed, Posilac-treated cows would give milk that was safe for humans to drink, and that the meat from those cows would be safe to eat. That cleared the path for Monsanto to find farmers to conduct field trials, which means that selected farmers around the country would try the drug on their own herds.

Many Americans trust the FDA to look out for their interests, to serve as a watchdog. So it may come as a surprise to some readers that the FDA's own laws require milk and meat from test herds to be sold to an unsuspecting public once the human health issues have been decided. The milk marketing cooperative to which Ken Nobis belongs, Michigan Milk Producers Association (MMPA), accepted the milk from the cows Ken used to test the drug. MMPA executives say that milk didn't go into the "fluid milk" supply—that's the milk that you and I buy in grocery stores in the plastic gallon jugs. It was routed instead into powdered milk, cheese, and butter production, products that the federal government buys as surplus.

That surplus food is given to this country's impoverished citizens, who count on the government's largesse to provide them with safe and wholesome food.

Monsanto consulted with MMPA in 1987, two years after the company had satisfied the FDA's human-health questions about the drug. Where, asked Monsanto, would MMPA prefer that test herds be located? And who would MMPA recommend as a farmer with good management practices? Who might be willing to help Monsanto test its drug?

MMPA officials thought of Ken, who had by then earned a dozen or so state dairy herd improvement awards. They spoke with Ken, who said he would consider testing the drug. He had done a similar test for Upjohn some years previously, when the Kalamazoo-based company was testing a conventionally produced synthetic hormone for dairy cows called prostaglandin, which is used to treat reproductive problems.

Part of the reason he felt comfortable working with Monsanto, Ken says, is because the company had hired a very highly regarded, newly retired Michigan State University dairy science professor, Dr. Bill Thomas. Thomas was to oversee Monsanto's on-farm tests; Ken knew Thomas from his work in dairy herd nutrition, and thought well of him, as do others around the world. All over the country Monsanto hired newly retired prominent dairy scientists as consultants; at universities across the nation Monsanto and the other chemical companies trying to develop their own versions of rBGH/rBST spent hundreds of thousands of dollars on grants for research conducted by still-active faculty at virtually every agricultural school there is. The drug companies routinely refer press questions about their versions of the drug to the nearest land-grant agricultural school; very often the person designated to answer questions about rBGH/rBST has spent years in drug company–funded research on the substance.

The hormone "wasn't a foreign idea to me," says Ken. "I knew something about BST then; I'd attended a couple of seminars at Michigan State University." In fact, the idea of a synthetic BST had been around since the '50s, when the hormone's existence and function were first discovered by scientists. And the dairy-industry press had been writing about BST and its bioengineered versions for more than a decade.

"Our first concern was, 'Does it adulterate the milk and meat?' " says Ken. "We were confident, based on the data that Monsanto had submitted to the FDA, that it does not."

The next concern was who would be responsible if the trial drug harmed or killed a cow. Monsanto promised Ken that it would pay for or replace any injured or killed cows, and the farmer and the company negotiated a reimbursement price. In the end the Nobises helped Monsanto test its drug in three trials.

The first began in December 1987, ending 120 days later. The test group was sixty cows. Thirty were treated with the drug—injected periodically with Posilac—and thirty went uninjected. Monsanto chose the cows and paired them by age, stage of lactation (where they were in the milk-making cycle), and levels of production. In this test, Monsanto employees injected the cows every fourteen days; the Nobises did not and were not to know which cows received the drug and which did not.

"We began to guess pretty soon, though," says Ken, "because those cows' production just went up a lot." Otherwise, he insists, the cows were indistinguishable: he saw no changes in their body weight or general appearance, no problems with feet or legs or reproductive cycles. Although critics of rBST/rBGH cite those and other problems as side effects of the bioengineered drugs, the Nobises saw nothing to make them wary of the drug.

As if by magic, however, the injected cows began to give more milk—an average of about eleven percent more. More milk is more profit for the dairyman, remember, and since the Nobises sold this milk through MMPA, their profits rose.

At the end of the first trial the cows were rested for thirty days, recalls Ken. Then the second trial began in April 1988.

This trial continued through the fall of 1990. In this trial Monsanto gave the Nobises a certain number of doses of the drug, enough to treat about 150 cows. The drug has no effect on a cow in its earliest stages of milk production, so it wouldn't be used on any cow before a certain date in its lactation cycle. And the drug has an effect for a fairly consistent number of days in the lactation cycle—too late, and its use does nothing to boost milk production.

But in this trial Monsanto didn't specify which cows to use the drug on, and they didn't tell the Nobises when to use the drug. "We were concerned about the drug's effect on conception rates," recalls Ken, "so we used it only on cows that were already confirmed pregnant or that were at least one hundred and eight days in milk. We didn't use it on any cows that were less than one hundred days in milk."

The test was successful, showing an approximate eight to twelve percent rise in milk production with no detriment to the cows that Ken could see. They "got the most bang for our buck" by beginning injections on cows that were about a third of the way into the three-hundred-day lactation cycle. And, says Ken, they noted in independent trials, separate of Monsanto's requirements, that the rBST/rBGH-treated cows required about five percent more feed than uninjected cows— but they didn't need different feed, just more of the same stuff they'd always eaten.

In the third test the Nobises began in November 1990 with a selection of 150 cows. In a test that lasted until January 1994 the Nobises monitored that group of cows for the kind of problems that cause a cow to be culled from the herd: reproductive problems, leg and foot problems, the udder infection called mastitis. Because this was a longevity trial to monitor the long-term effects of the drug on cows injected with it, the Nobises didn't move cows into and out of the test group.

They found that the percentage of cows treated with Monsanto's bioengineered rBST/rBGH that were culled from the herd because of mastitis was lower than the cull rate for their untreated cows. "We never babied them," Ken says. "We've never had a separate group of treated animals. They've always been mixed in with the rest of the cows. And we didn't feed different rations to the test animals."

They saw only one injection-site abscess—another of the critics' complaints about the drug—in the cows they treated. "That was when we still used the same needle to inject all the cows," he says. "We never had the problem again when we switched to one cow, one needle." That is perhaps why Monsanto offers Posilac in premeasured doses in disposable needles, which the company wants returned for proper disposal.

"We're skeptics," says Ken. "We scrutinized our cows closer than most people would have for herd health. We didn't have a single problem with Posilac."

Ken says Monsanto didn't pay him to test the drug, that his incentive was "free product (Posilac) from 1987 to 1993, and the profits from the extra milk we sold."

But he adds that "the most we ever added to our herd average was twenty-five hundred pounds—about a twelve percent increase." And he says that other dairy management techniques—separating the cows into groups of roughly the same age, and improved feeding methods—may have contributed to that rise in milk production. "It's difficult to measure the response rate for BST," he says.

But through all three tests, Ken asserts that they saw no problems with the cows injected with Monsanto's drug. No matter what the critics say about this drug, Ken can say only positive things about Posilac. His cows had no problems with rBST/rBGH. None. Never.

## MILLIONS FOR RESEARCH—AND MILLIONS
## FOR MARKETING

Monsanto's marketing department put together a little information kit for dairy farmers, ready to be shipped as soon as the FDA gave its approval to Posilac. Virtually every dairy farmer in the country received a copy of the kit, which is an impressive bit of business, after the FDA approved Posilac in November 1993. Each kit includes a booklet discussing Posilac in glowing terms, a voucher good for $150 in veterinary services—about which more in the next chapter—and a videotape entitled *A Good Producer's Introduction to Posilac.*

Ken Nobis is featured in the video quite prominently. He speaks more often than any of the other farmers who appear, and whenever he speaks he looks off up into the heavens to the left of his head. His parts of the video were filmed on a balmy summer day on his farm; he wears a short-sleeved plaid cotton shirt, and his hair is neatly combed with a sharp part on the left side.

The five-minute video is narrated mostly by an avuncular man in his middle fifties who wears blue jeans and a red flannel shirt open at the throat. He tells us that Posilac is "the single most tested product in history"—curiously, the same claim Calgene has made for its bioengineered tomato—which he holds as proof of its safety and merit. "Of course, you'll want to inject Posilac in every eligible cow," says the unidentified narrator, "as every cow not treated is a lost income opportunity."

Over and over again the narrator stresses how easy it is to use Posilac, how quick and simple it is for the farmer to inject his cows. "You can see how easy the injections are," he says cheerily to the viewer, and he says so at least three times. The narrator's insistent refrain is backed up by dairyman Jeff True of Wyoming County, New York. A thirtyish farmer with an open, honest face, True says Posilac is right for him to use on his farm, and it's ever so easy to use: "One person can do fifty cows in twenty minutes." Later in the video, True will remind the viewer that "any response I get [from injecting Posilac] is profit in my pocket."

Colorado dairyman Mike Dickinson from Larimer County checks in, too, again telling the viewer that Posilac is simple to use. He says he saw an average increase of ten pounds of milk a day from the cows he injected with Posilac. Any dairyman would be foolish not to use it, he seems to imply, telling us that "BST is not any different than artificial insemination was—it's a herd management tool."

One of Ken's sound bites affirms that as well, and in our conversation he will repeat this opinion. But in the video Ken also reassures a viewing farmer that he won't have to do much different in the way of feeding his cows. Cows that produce lots of milk need lots of feed, says Ken, but it's just a matter of making sure the ration already in use is always there for the cow to eat.

To a nonfarmer there is something chilling about this video. It's not the footage of farmhands, both male and female, moving down the lines of cows injecting them with the drug at the bases of their tails; they could be injecting vitamins or antibiotics or any number of other things. Some of the cows flinch at the injections, some do not. Nor is it the cheerleading of the narrator and all the farmers who consented to take part in the video's production; these are farmers who tested Posilac for Monsanto, after all, and the narrator is no doubt a hired gun.

No, what's chilling about this video is its bloodless business approach to the science of modern dairying. There are dozens of cows in almost every segment, but no one ever touches them—except to inject them. Cows are shown eating in long rows stretching to the camera's horizon; cows are shown in milking parlors, but you have to look closely to recognize them from that angle as the creatures they are. There are cows in barns, but no cows in pastures. That's not how cows are "managed" these days.

And remember: "Every eligible cow left untreated is a lost income opportunity."

We've come full circle on the farm tour. Back in the office now, Ken and I draw to the end of our visit. He says he doesn't understand why consumers have any concerns at all about this drug. It is safe, and a lot of important people have agreed on that: the American Medical Association, the National Institutes of Health, the American Dietetic Association have all joined the FDA in assuring the public that rBST/rBGH poses no threat to consumers. When I mention that I find it interesting that Monsanto gave the American Dietetic Association about $100,000 to fund ADA's rBST/rBGH consumer hotline—an act that in my view seriously tarnishes ADA's reputation—Ken seems surprised. "They did?" he says.

Still, he says, consumer worries about this heavily tested hormone are tantamount to an insistence on a risk-free world—an unfeasible proposition. It's none of the consumer's business how he produces milk as long as he's following the law and maintaining purity, he says with surprising ferocity. "It's people like you," he says to me, meaning the media, "who have stirred up the consumers, making them afraid of this stuff." There are no food safety issues for the American public to be concerned about, he says, just television and newspaper reporters who want to get viewers or sell advertising. I ask Ken about reports of salmonella on raw chicken and in eggs, about *E. coli* contamination in beef. Doesn't the public have a right to know about those things, I ask. He is silent.

We must agree to disagree, I say. I have some questions about rBST/rBGH that remain unanswered by the experts, just as I have some questions about the way food is produced in this country in general and its effects on our environment. Ken begins to shake his head before I finish speaking. There is no environmental crisis in this country, he says. "I see more deer on this farm than we ever did when I was a kid. When my dad saw a deer in one of the fields, it was a big event, something we talked about over dinner. It's the same thing with ducks and geese. And look at Lake Erie—it's come back almost completely. We're doing a great job with the environment, but nobody ever writes about that. Instead, they write about all the things that are supposed to be going wrong."

What people like me don't understand, he says, people who want to buy a house in the country and then don't like the smells of the farms they wanted as their neighbors, is this: "Production efficiency equals more production at a lower cost."

"We approach it from many angles," says Ken, who is by now fairly passionate in tone and temper. "You can only handle so many cows per person. The production cost is the same per cow. It's going to cost $750 for each stall in a new barn, whether the stalls are filled with low producers or high producers."

Why not be sure those expensive stalls are filled with high producers?

As politely as possible, I tell Ken that I understand his perspective, but I simply do not share his views. It has been a long day, and we are both a little vexed by the frustrations of trying, truly trying, to understand someone who thinks in a totally different way.

He has been patient with me, and he has been forthright in answering every question I've put to him. My sense of Ken Nobis is that he is a proud and stubborn man, a man who is not used to impudent visitors who question his rightness.

I have spent a full day—from ten a.m. to nearly five p.m.
—with Ken, touring his farm and struggling to understand the
way he approaches his life's work.

In that time he has offered me neither food nor drink. He
has not offered water or coffee or doughnut or sandwich.

And neither has he taken any himself.

*5*

# One Man Can Milk Just
# Fifty Cows

*D*avid McCartney never wanted to be anything but a dairy farmer. He grew up among cows, the fourth generation on this family farm outside Coleman, Michigan, wanting nothing more than to turn his hand to dairying. He dreamed of cows of his own.

But the shy, blond, twenty-eight-year-old with the slight stammer had some powerful obstacles to overcome before he could put the milker on his first holstein.

McCartney and his wife, dark-haired, pretty, twenty-six-year-old Lynda Jackson McCartney, have worked harder than most of their peers to achieve their dream. For a while, early in their four-year marriage, they each worked two full-time jobs: he worked at Ittner Bean and Grain, the local grain elevator, and tended to the McCartneys' calves and farm whenever he wasn't working at the elevator; Lynda worked at the library at Central Michigan University in nearby Mount Pleasant, as well as holding down a job as a sign language interpreter and tutor for a seventh-grade student in the Clare public schools, somewhat farther away. The couple lived on his pay from the grain elevator, banking all of Lynda's pay. They were saving.

Saving to buy more cows.

We are seated in the McCartneys' dining room at the aging table with the mismatched chairs. We have just had a farmer's dinner, a main meal in the middle of the day: steaks from the freezer; some home-grown green beans, also from the freezer; scalloped potatoes and bread sticks; and a pitcher of milk, unpasteurized and unhomogenized, from that morning's milking of the McCartneys' own cows. I have been making a fool of myself over this milk. I have drunk two glasses already and am wondering if I would be remiss in pouring myself another.

David grew up in this house. He sits in the same seat that he took at every meal through his childhood, he and his three sisters and his parents all coming to this table day after day after day. The house looks as if it could use a little updating; my hunch is that this wallpaper, here in the dining room, is the same wallpaper he saw as a child.

But the sense of this house isn't in its decor. It is, instead, in David and Lynda's obvious, deep, unshakable belief in each other and in their dreams.

David McCartney, the fourth-generation farmer, and his wife, who grew up a "town girl," the daughter of a truck-driving father and a teaching mother, will not be dissuaded by the experts who tell them they can't farm the way they are, in fact, farming.

The McCartneys milk about thirty holsteins on their 118-acre farm, and they are well on the way to making their farm a certified organic enterprise. To understand what an achievement that is, one has to understand the intricacies of milk marketing, and that is a topic that even experts have a hard time explaining. The way milk gets to your supermarket dairy case—and the byzantine maze of state and federal regulations underpinning the system—warrant a moment's study.

Far and away the most common breed of dairy cow you'll see today is the holstein-friesian, the black-and-white beauties that dot the landscape in everyone's mental picture of bucolic peacefulness. Holsteins have come to be the breed of choice for most dairymen, displacing the jerseys and guernseys and Brown Swiss that used to be more common, because holsteins are high-volume producers, placid, and their milk is higher in protein, lower in butterfat. Those last two qualities mean more profit for the farmer, whose milk profits are based on both quantity and quality. He'll get a premium for high protein, which is important for cheese-makers and other processors; he gets a premium for milk that has a certain percentage, usually about 3.5 percent of butterfat. A holstein's milk, generally, is right about 3.5 percent. Milk from jerseys, by comparison, is closer to 4.5 percent butterfat.

Holsteins give a lot of milk in just the right composition for a dairyman to get the most return on his investment of time, energy, and labor. Careful breeding has brought forth generations of cows that can produce thirty thousand pounds of milk a year or more, although most dairy farmers' herds don't include these blue-ribbon producers.

Think of that for a moment. Thirty thousand pounds of milk a year: that's about eighty-two pounds of milk a day averaged over the entire year; more than forty pounds of milk every milking, morning and evening. Although farmers sell milk by the hundredweight, we usually think of milk in the form that we buy it: by the gallon. So, since a gallon of milk weighs 8.75 pounds, you might think of that prize-winning cow's milk production this way: nearly ten gallons of milk every day of the year.

But think, too, of this. At my favorite market a gallon of whole milk, when it's not on special, sells for just over $2.25. I'd pay about $22.50 for all the milk one of these well-bred holsteins could produce in a single day.

The farmer who fed, sheltered, and milked that cow, however, wouldn't earn even half that much. His reward for his labors could be as little as $8.78, total, for that cow's one-day milk production. He might get $3,000 or more a year from the milk each top-producing cow in his herd produces. Of course, the farmer has to subtract the cost of the cow's feed, bedding, and medicines; the cost of utilities and gas to run the farm machinery; and other operating expenses. And, of course, that $3,000 would come from only the highest-producing cow.

Part of the reason the farmer's return is so different from the price you pay is that two federal programs regulate dairy prices.

The first is the Marketing Order Program, established in the 1930s. It sets the price that milk processors—we'll talk about them in a  moment—must pay farmers. The aim of that Depression-era program was to raise farmers' incomes, to provide a steady, adequate milk supply, and to promote orderly marketing.

The Marketing Order Program doesn't work, though, when there's a surplus of milk and processors aren't eager to buy it.

So in 1949 the federal government began the dairy price support program. Under this program the federal government buys all unsold processed milk products. Because fluid milk, the kind we buy to drink, has a limited shelf life, surpluses are routinely turned into more long-lived staples like cheese, butter, and milk powder.

The government uses taxpayers' money to buy these products; they are given to lower-income citizens. These products are what are described as "butter mountains" and "cheese stockpiles" tucked away in government storehouses.

From 1952 to 1972 the dairy support program cost taxpayers an average of $325 million a year. But by 1979 the government began to spend upward of $1 billion each year. By 1982–83 the government was spending more than $2.5 billion of taxpayers' money to buy surplus dairy products. As you can see, in the forty-five years since the federal government began the dairy price support program, there has never been a shortage of milk and milk products in this country.

The federal government responded to the high cost of the dairy price support program in 1982–83 in two ways under the 1985 farm bill.

First, it ordered a voluntary government buyout of many dairy farmers: you may remember seeing photos and television reports of hundreds of thousands of dairy cows being slaughtered around the country. The idea and its logic are reasonably self-evident: fewer cows meant less surplus for the government to purchase.

The government also changed the formula for calculating dairy price supports. The new formula contained two key figures: if the government expected to buy more than 5 billion pounds of milk the following year, prices would *drop* by fifty cents per hundredweight, but if the government expected to buy fewer than 2.5 billion pounds, the price would *rise* by fifty cents.

In 1987 the milk support price was $11.35 per hundredweight. In 1990 it fell to $10.10.

The 1990 farm bill kept the milk support price of $10.10; that price is a floor, which is to say that the prices may go higher but they may not go lower. But the 1990 farm bill also empowered the secretary of agriculture to impose a special assessment on all dairy farmers—high producers and low—if the government buys more than seven billion pounds of milk products in a year. In the 1990 federal budget Congress enacted an additional assessment for overproduction that essentially reduced the price paid to a farmer by 5 cents per hundredweight in 1990, and by 11.25 cents per hundredweight in the years 1992 through 1995 if the farmer increases his production.

The short-term fall in milk production after the government's buyout and slaughter of dairy cattle didn't last long; improved breeding made production per cow increasingly higher, and before long, milk production was back at virtually pre-buyout levels.

Curiously enough, milk prices for you and me at the supermarket have risen dramatically since 1985; the average price of a half-gallon of milk rose from $1.11 in 1985 to $1.43 in 1990—an increase of nearly thirty percent in five years.

The dairy farmer is caught in a double bind. His profits are linked to the volume of milk he can sell; in theory, the more milk he can wring from his cows, the more money he should make. But he is penalized if his production is too high, because the federal government has little interest in buying and stockpiling still more surplus dairy products.

Yet you and I continue to pay ever higher prices for milk and other dairy products at market. It defies the logic of supply and demand, but there you have it.

The key to the difference in what the farmer earns and what we pay may be found at any of several doorsteps.

Few dairymen sell directly to a processor—a company that bottles milk, for example, and sells it to your supermarket under its own label or under the label of a store or a national brand. And few sell directly to manufacturers such as cheese factories.

Instead, most dairymen belong to a dairy cooperative. These organizations,, working on behalf of their member farmers, accept the milk from the farm, test it for purity and quality, and sell it in bulk to processors. When the processor pays the co-op for the milk, the co-op pays the farmer for his share of the sale. When a farmer speaks of his milk check, he's talking about the checks he gets from his co-op—you might say they're a farmer's paychecks, although the farmer is not an employee of the co-op.

The milk from several farms is blended in the tank truck, driven by an independent milk hauler, as the truck makes its way along its daily route. The farmer pays the hauler who picks up his milk, but it wouldn't look like that if you saw the farmer's milk check: the co-op deducts hauling charges, at rates privately negotiated by hauler and farmer, from the farmer's milk checks, and the co-op writes the check to the hauler.

Co-ops function differently in different dairy states. In Wisconsin, for example, dozens of co-ops exist, and competition among them is fierce. A Wisconsin dairyman may have a choice among a half-dozen co-ops who all want him as a member; he may change co-ops one or several times a year, depending on price, pickup routes, and a variety of other factors. Some of the co-ops pride themselves on serving only organic dairymen; others offer slightly better prices or various other incentives to the farmer who's trying to make the most of his investment. This is true, too, in California, which recently surpassed Wisconsin as the largest dairy state; in Minnesota; and in Vermont.

In Michigan, the fifth-largest dairy state, the situation is different. Far and away the largest dairy co-op in the state is

Michigan Milk Producers Association, with some three thousand members as of 1992; the next largest co-op has only eight hundred members. In Michigan if you are a dairyman who doesn't want to sign the one-year contract that MMPA requires of its members, your milk may go unsold. Milk isn't a commodity like corn or wheat that can be held back from the market if prices are low; the dairy farmer is caught here, too: he has to sell his perishable product to make room for the next day's milking, and the next, and the next.

When I was a child in rural Jackson County, Michigan, the stainless-steel tanker trucks picking up milk were a familiar sight on the back roads outside our village, the roads that led to my classmates' family farms. They are less common now, since so many of those farms have gone out of business, but you still see them on county roads and highways.

The system has some oddities. A small artisanal cheese company in Ann Arbor buys milk from a nearby dairy; the milk is picked up at the farm and delivered directly to the cheese dairy, but the cheesemakers buy the milk from MMPA, even though the milk never passes through the doors of the co-op's plant, because the farmer has signed a contract with MMPA.

And there are still, in Michigan, a handful of dairies who milk their own cows and bottle their own milk. Some still deliver to the house, bringing the milk in returnable glass bottles; others offer their own milk for sale in stores on their farms, or sell it wholesale to local grocery stores. There may be dairies like that in your state, too, although they are ever rarer; the economics of the dairy industry together with the avalanche of state and federal laws regulating dairying makes it harder and harder for these small enterprises to make a go of it.

But in most cases, if I buy milk at a Michigan grocery store, it's MMPA milk, whether it's labeled Kroger or Borden or Farm Fresh or Sealtest or Meadowbrook or Detroit City Dairy. That will most likely be true in your state as well. No matter what the label says, it's locally produced milk, probably sold to a processor by a local dairy farmers' co-op.

It is the co-op and the processor who, between them, set the price that the farmer receives for the milk he works so hard to produce. And it is the processor—and the processor's clients—who set the prices that you and I will pay for milk at the supermarket.

Understanding all that, you may wonder why David and Lynda McCartney have made it their lives' work to dairy farm.

"For me, it's being a steward of God's land," says Lynda, thinking carefully and choosing her words slowly. "We are charged with making this land productive, to feed us and the animals."

Her pragmatic husband nods in agreement but adds some further reasons of his own. "It's the independence and the challenge of working alone," he says. "There's a freedom in taking responsibility for all this. If things go right, the rewards are mine; if things go wrong, the responsibility is mine."

Pragmatic he is, but still daft about cows: "And one of the biggest thrills is when a cow has a calf. It's just the neatest thing in the world to watch and be part of. It's real hard for me to tear myself away when a cow is calving: I just want to stay and watch the miracle."

There was only one road to adulthood for David, and like the yellow brick road in *The Wizard of Oz*, it would eventually lead him back home.

"When I was in high school I rented seventy acres to plant cash crops," he says, remembering those days with evident pride. "When I graduated from high school in 1984,

I knew I wanted to farm. But my parents really discouraged me."

His father was still dairy farming then, his mother still teaching in the Coleman public schools. But his father was beginning to think about retiring; with years of experience in dairy farming, seeing the diminishing fortune of the dairy farmer, he thought it no place for his young son.

"I worked for nothing for my dad for two years," recalls David, "but then finally I had to start getting paid. My dad turned the cows over to me, and I began managing the farm in 1986—just in time for disaster. It rained for twenty-eight consecutive days in September of 1986, an inch or more every day. Thirty inches of rain that month! It took out three hundred acres of sorghum, oats, corn, and hay. We were able to buy grain, and we bought hay from a neighbor. But it was tough."

David remembers 1987 as a good year, 1988 as a drought: "Two bad years out of three," he says with a natural-born farmer's acceptance of—and frustration with—the things he can't control.

His father and his grandfather had attended Michigan State University's well-regarded agricultural programs, and David thought it prudent to follow in their footsteps. He didn't think it necessary to enroll in a full four-year dairy science program, which would have given him a bachelor of science degree and aimed him along the route of research or work with an agricultural company. Instead, in 1987, while managing the farm, he enrolled in the two-year dairy production program—a working farmer's training program teaching the most up-to-date ideas about dairying.

But by this time his dad didn't want the cows back, he says, rubbing the back of his neck. He had deeded them all to David and wanted to retire. So for the first year David rose at four a.m., went out to milk, feed, and settle the cows,

showered, and dressed on his way down to East Lansing—
seventy-five miles each way. He'd be there in time for an
eight o'clock class, be in school all day, then drive back,
milk again, eat, and fall asleep. "I got to be pretty good at
dressing in the car, and I got so I could do the trip each way
in about an hour—probably I shouldn't have, but I had to,"
he says.

Finally, in 1988 he made a difficult decision: he would
sell the thirty cows, both to ease his schedule and to raise
the money he needed for school. He also sold "about three-
quarters of the machinery and the silos," David says, but he
didn't sell the farm. His parents, meanwhile, had built a new
house on a small parcel from the farm.

The certificate that David earned at MSU is framed
and hangs over his old small desk, its cubbyholes overflow-
ing with paperwork, which is tucked into one corner of
the dining room. He is proud of the certificate, and hearing
the story of how it was earned, I can't blame him: I know
no one, including myself, who worked so hard to earn an
academic credential.

Unfortunately, the decision to sell the cows created some
new problems for the young dairyman.

"When I came back I thought it would be easy to start
milking again," he says. "But I found out I had forty years'
worth of improvements to make. The Michigan Department
of Agriculture would allow a lot of things if they were grand-
fathered, but they wanted them fixed if I was going to start a
new dairy."

Undeterred, David went to work for the grain elevator,
where he earned $4 an hour—and watched his neighbors
spend hundreds of thousands of dollars on agricultural chemicals. "Working for $4 an hour—that changed my attitude
some," he says. "I knew then that that wasn't what I wanted.
And I couldn't believe these guys coming in. They were

spending more money than I'd make in a year, on fertilizers and pesticides and stuff. They'd be grumbling about it all the time, but they'd do it."

Little by little, David began to figure some things out. He realized that the schooling he'd worked so hard to finish had not prepared him to farm productively, but had instead taught him how to be a customer of the agro-chemical companies. He began to see the men who spent such vast amounts of money on chemical products going out of business—and not understanding why. He began to think that the key to successful farming might lie not in productivity but in prudence.

"The farmer gets the same line of advice from everyone," he says. "It comes from the university, from the extension agent, from the seed companies, even from the elevator staff. They all say the same thing: the stress is on productivity. You have to produce more, always more—and always more than your neighbors."

And so this hardheaded young man who wouldn't give up began to think about dairying in some new ways. "Between forty and sixty percent of a farm's gross income goes to feeding the cows, what with growing grain, buying and maintaining the equipment to plant and reap the grain, etc. That's a twenty percent difference right there—and that difference could make or break a farm in a bad year," he says.

Drawn to the idea of organic farming because of his feelings of good stewardship for the land, David slowly rethought everything he'd learned from some of the leading dairy experts in the country. Some of what he learned was good, he decided; he kept that. But much of it was useless, and that he discarded, trusting in his own instincts.

"At MSU, they say no-till (a method of field management where the soil is not plowed every year) saves time and energy, and you're not losing the soil to wind erosion. Using no-till, it cost me $88 an acre to grow corn, when I figured in the seed, the fertilizer, and the chemicals; that's compared to about $100 an acre for the neighbors—one of whom has since gone out of business."

That was a good saving, David thought, but he kept thinking.

He realized that he could plant sorghum, plow in his cows' manure, skip the fertilizers, and just pay for the seed. That brought his costs down to about $40 an acre. "See?" he says. "The key isn't necessarily productivity: it's profitability. And the way we farm—the way we're taught to farm—costs a lot of money, which means it's harder for the farmer to make money."

By 1992, now married and with the many repairs on the barns finished, David and Lynda bought nine cows from a neighbor to add to the three they'd raised from calves. They started milking with just a dozen cows and borrowed enough money to buy another dozen about two months later.

He has stopped growing grain for his cows, finding it more cost-effective to buy the little he needs; his cows graze in open pasture, in a return to an older style of herd management called rotational grazing. The cows are moved from field to field every few weeks, and they get most of their nourishment from pasture for more than nine months a year. He buys no fertilizers, pesticides, or herbicides since he doesn't have to worry about high yields on grain crops for feed; and he rarely needs to administer antibiotics for mastitis, the udder infection common in high-producing cows; upper respiratory problems in calves; and abscesses and swellings. Because his cows depend barely at all on commercial feeds, they don't get subtherapeutic doses of antibiotics in their meals.

He's happy with his cows' milk production, David says,

and he doesn't need to push it higher and higher to offset higher and higher costs. David just wants to milk cows for his living. He doesn't want to own so many cows that he has to hire a flock of employees to help him tend them.

## *DAVID VS. GOLIATH*

When Monsanto launched Posilac in February 1994, it was nearly frantic to begin recouping its multimillion-dollar investment in the drug. It invited dairy farmers to take advantage of a "special introductory price" of just $6 a dose, and as of July of that year, that price was still offered. Periodic rumors swept through dairy states that the company was even giving the drug away, although the rumors were impossible to confirm.

Offering veterinary vouchers worth $150 to every farmer who ordered Posilac through the toll-free Monsanto phone number was a shrewd marketing move on Monsanto's part, albeit a risky one. Contemporary dairy farmers view their veterinarians as near-partners, not just doctors for sick animals, and the voucher was meant to allay concerns about the drug's side effects. In fact, some veterinarians in many states decided they wouldn't accept the vouchers for fear that problems that might appear down the road would make them as liable as the drug company for damages, both to beasts and humans.

While the FDA and Monsanto continued to insist that Posilac was safe for cows and humans, the federal General Accounting Office continued to hold its position that mastitis problems in rBST/rBGH–treated cows had not been adequately explored by the FDA or the drug companies. The GAO also expressed concerns, as did a number of other scientists and social activists, about dangers to humans, especially children, posed by another hormone, Insulin-like Growth

Factor 1 (IGF-1). Bovine growth hormone is not believed to be active in humans, and is, in fact, chemically different in structure from its human counterpart. But both bovine and human somatotropin produce rises in IGF-1, which is linked to development problems in humans, and IGF-1 in cows and humans *is* chemically identical. Since Monsanto has essentially stopped funding research on rBST/rBGH—the 1994 annual meeting of the American Dairy Science Association didn't even list bovine somatotropin on its convention discussion list—these questions remain unanswered.

Meanwhile, the FDA released a very stringent set of guidelines for dairy processors who wished to label their milk as rBST/rBGH–free; essentially, the watchdog agency took the very unusual position that even dairy farms that process their own milk had to use a disclaimer that stated that there is no known difference between milk from treated and untreated cows. Monsanto seized on the FDA's ruling as adequate grounds to file suit against two dairies, Brown Swiss Dairies in Iowa and the Pure Milk and Ice Cream Company of Waco, Texas. (Both suits were eventually settled out of court.) The company charged that the two dairies' labels endangered its ability to recoup its investment in Posilac, an arguably shaky legal leg since there is little legal precedent that consumers have a responsibility to help business recover investments in research. Both dairies had used the FDA "suggested wording" exactly as the agency issued it on their labels. Although there seemed little chance that Monsanto could win these suits, given that the dairies followed the letter of the law, many dairy farmers around the country thought they understood Monsanto's motives. Dare to label your milk rBST/rBGH–free, the suits seemed to say, and we'll entangle you in a long, very expensive legal battle. The drug company may not win the suits, but for dairy farmers that hardly matters: the cost of defending themselves against such a suit would put many, if not most, small dairy farmers out of business.

The FDA is not allowed under federal law to consider social and economic issues when it approves a drug; its only concerns, by law, are efficacy—does the drug do what it purports to do?—and safety for human and beast.

But dozens of other agencies have considered rBST/rBGH's impact on the family dairy farmer, and none of the studies have presented rosy news for farmers like David McCartney.

A 1990 poll conducted by the National Dairy Board—commissioned as part of a $1 million public relations campaign by NDB to convince consumers that there is no problem with rBST/rBGH in milk—found nearly half of the shoppers surveyed would reduce their dairy consumption if they knew the drug was used. Only a third of the people surveyed by NDB said they trusted the FDA's assurances that rBST/rBGH was safe.

A grassroots coalition of small dairy farmers, Family Farm Defenders, was angered by NDB's pro-growth hormone stance and its million-dollar public relations campaign. Family Farm Defenders petitioned the United States Department of Agriculture to hold a referendum on whether to end NDB's mandatory-checkoff funding—money farmers must pay to NDB, whether they support the promotion board's positions or not—in 1993 and again in 1994. The difference in the number of signatures required for the petitions to be approved—in the span of one year—dropped by some fifteen percent. Fifteen percent of the country's dairy farmers had gone out of business in a single year, according to the Department of Agriculture's own statistics. That was before rBST/rBGH was approved, said Family Farm Defenders; the coalition fears rBST/rBGH will drive even more dairy families from their farms.

And by the summer of 1994, dairy trade papers and small-town rural weekly newspapers carried a number of virtually unthinkable ads: dairy farmers selling off their herds in the middle of the summer, when they stood to lose the most money, when their grain crops were already in the ground.

A 1991 study on biotechnology conducted by the federal Office of Technology Assessment (OTA) predicted "a mass exodus" in small- to moderate-sized dairy farms over the next five to fifteen years as the result of rBST/rBGH use. The Northeast and the Great Lakes states would see the largest loss of family farms, the study predicted, since most dairy farmers in these regions have 50 to 150 cows. Two Cornell University agricultural economists, J. Sellschopp and R. J. Kalter, also surmised in a 1989 study that rBST/rBGH adoption would be highest in areas with larger average herd sizes—California, as compared to Vermont, for example—because of "advantages in management, technical information, and risk evaluation."

Monsanto and the other drug companies have argued that rBST/rBGH is a tool that levels the playing field in the dairy industry, as it were. It is relatively inexpensive, the companies say, and is therefore feasible for any dairy farmer, no matter how large or small his herd, to use.

The economic impact studies don't bear that out, precisely. What they say, instead, is that rBST/rBGH will contribute to a flood of milk in this country—and that the losers, when milk prices drop as a result of that gigantic surplus, will be farmers who can least afford to compete against bigger dairies.

Farmers precisely like David McCartney.

One of the calves in David's pen has taken a liking to the wooden button on my heavy sweater and is determined to chew it off. I bat at its head gently, trying to dissuade it, but its determination is remarkable. In the end, all I can do is turn my hip to the creature and rub the poll of its head, which seems to please it.

David laughs. "They're real nosy," he says, wading through the calves to rescue me and my sweater. He rubs each calf himself, briefly, as he pushes them aside.

In the small milking parlor of his grandfather's barn, David's radio chatters. It's an old radio, hung on a nail, and it's tuned to a talk-radio station. He turns it off, coloring high on the cheeks as if caught in some embarrassing act. "It's kind of lonesome out here in the early morning," he says. "The cows and I, we like to listen to the news together."

His cows are milked side by side, in a half-dozen or so stanchions, metal devices that clasp loosely around the cows' necks to steady them in one spot. It takes him a couple of hours to get them all milked and everything all cleaned up afterward, he says, and I think of how raw it must be out here at six o'clock in the morning on a winter day, when the snow lies thick and deep around the barns as it does today.

But I have been in barns like this at morning milking, and I know, too, that there is an ineffable peace in those hours. I know that David will speak softly to his cows as he milks them, that they will mutter to themselves and to him in response. I know the sound of the swish of cows' tails, and the sound of their teeth as they chew their grain. The barn will be sweet with the smell of hay and of the cows themselves, rich with the earthy scent of their dung.

I can feel that David softens when he is around his cows, that his breath slows and his pace drops. This is where he is happiest, I believe, and this is all he wants from life: to greet his cows twice each day, every day for as long as he is able, and to take from them what they will give at their own pace.

It is a modest enough dream. And an imperiled one.

# 6

# *A Chicken for 212,400 Pots Every Week*

*W*hen Jim Pastore Sr. talks about chicken, it makes sense to listen: he's been in the poultry business for nearly half a century, beginning in 1946 at the age of fourteen when he and his father operated a "dressed-while-you-wait" poultry shop in Canton, Ohio. Housewives came to the store and chose the chicken they wanted; Pastore employees killed and plucked the birds while the buyers waited, the customers often watching intently to make sure the bird they took home was the one they'd picked out.

Those days are long past for the sixty-two-year-old Jim, though, lost in part because a road expansion in 1954 made it difficult for customers to get to the store. At about the same time, he says, the housewives who had patronized the shop began to prefer to buy their chicken from the new ultramodern supermarkets, where everything they needed in their weekly shopping was available under one roof. In those stores, the chicken came already cut up and neatly wrapped; it was the beginning of a generation of American shoppers who could forget that the chicken they ate came from a live bird—like the woman who couldn't tell chicken skin from plastic wrap.

Shops like Jim's looked old-fashioned and dated by comparison with the brightly lit, gleaming superstores. Today, the few remaining such poultry shops—usually located in large cities, where their clientele is predominantly ethnic—struggle to survive. Jim says he doubts those in operation now will remain profitable long enough for their owners to pass them on to their own sons and daughters.

Since then the poultry business has changed immensely, Jim says from his modestly opulent office at Park Farms headquarters, built on the site of his father's poultry shop. Today, Park Farms is the smallest integrated broiler operation in the country, a fact that seems to amuse the no-nonsense Jim: "We're fifty-fourth out of fifty-four," he says, chuckling.

Chickens are raised for two reasons in this country, and the two no longer overlap. Broiler chickens are what you buy cut up at the supermarket, often on special for prices so low that one dollar will buy a whole bird weighing as much as four pounds. Broilers are also the birds from which come the ocean of boneless, skinless chicken breasts that flood into fast-food operations and school lunchrooms for chicken nuggets, so many chicken breasts that the leftover legs are very often a far better buy, selling for cents-per-pound, rather than dollars. "If we could figure out how to breed a chicken without legs and with four breasts," another poultryman once said to me, only half kidding, "we'd do it in a heartbeat."

But broiler chickens are not used to produce eggs; the chickens that lay eggs for our consumption are entirely different breeds, bred for different characteristics and raised in a different way. It is almost as if humans had created two entirely different races of chicken to suit their needs.

It wasn't always so. Traditionally, a flock of chickens was the farmwife's responsibility, and butter-and-egg money made it possible for her to buy the sundries she wanted or needed to see her household run smoothly. She sold any surplus eggs, and when old hens stopped laying, they went into the stew pot. In fact, the phrase "spring chicken" doesn't refer to the barely six-week-old chickens we buy today; it describes a poult—a young chicken that hasn't begun laying yet—hatched the previous summer. It was because the farmwife saw her chickens' value largely in the eggs they laid that a chicken in every pot was considered a luxury before World War II. No prudent farmwife would casually kill the birds she counted on to give her a salable foodstuff. Broilers, to that farmwife, were extra young roosters, slaughtered before they became fully grown and aggressive—and tough.

Even would-be farmers who buy chicks by mail today find their choices laid out by type of bird; most poultry catalogs offer breeds that are good layers or good meat birds, but few choices exist for a dual-purpose bird.

It is laying hens that are kept in small cages for their entire lives, standing on wire mesh floors and producing an egg or more each day for most of their productive lives. Laying hens are also often debeaked as chicks, which is to say the tips of their beaks are burned away so they can't peck at their neighbors. And when laying hens no longer lay, their carcasses are sold for livestock and pet foods, or to canneries that put out chicken stock and soup. It is a rare occurrence to see stewing hens at the supermarket these days, but that is how an exhausted laying hen would be labeled if one made it to your store.

Broilers, by contrast, are reared in low-roofed sheds, mostly in the South for several reasons, as we will see. Eighteen thousand chicks or more are raised in the same shed, their water and feed delivered by automatic, computer-controlled systems. Most modern broiler farms have several such sheds. It is said that these chicks are so perfectly bred and trained that they will starve themselves to death if water and food are placed on the ground, where chickens traditionally hunted and pecked for bugs and grain, rather than in the elevated troughs from which they are trained to feed.

At first, when the birds are small, the shed's partitions shorten their usable space, crowding the chicks together to help them keep warm and to make it easier for the poultryman to feed and water them. Later, as they grow, the partitions will be removed until at last the whole long, low shed is aswarm with birds. All are theoretically free to move about the entire shed, but in fact that doesn't really happen much: chickens subscribe to the social network called pecking order, and most birds will spend their lives within a few feet of where they first lit as chicks.

Modern breeding has changed the way these chickens look, too. Since feathers just get in the way in killing and dressing and don't offer the grower much in the way of profit, these contemporary chickens are bedraggled creatures, their feathers sparse and scanty. You won't find a chicken that looks anything like your notion of what a chicken should look like, breasty and proud, in this country's broiler grow-out operations.

Jim is one of the owners of Park Farms, but he and his family hold a controlling interest of only 55 percent of the company's shares. Employees own the balance, he says, and their interest is seen everywhere, a tangible pride evident even in the packing room, which we will visit later.

The company sells its labeled chicken within a 150-mile radius of Canton, selling directly to retailers or to packing houses, which function as distributors. While Park Farms is nowhere near as large as industry leader Tyson Foods, Inc.— which is the world's largest broiler producer and the largest manufacturer of value-added chicken nuggets—its organization mimics that of the larger companies, and we should learn how that system works.

We will learn about it from Jim because he is one of the few poultry processors left in this country who is not afraid to talk to reporters. Tyson, Perdue, and Holly Farms executives all declined to be interviewed for this book; they view the media with a great deal of suspicion since stories about salmonella in raw chicken and eggs have been brought to the public eye. They still wince from stories touted by animal rights groups about the crowded, perhaps inhumane, living conditions for the chickens in the sheds.

Before World War II, as we have seen, chicken-rearing was a job for women and children on the farm. But after the war researchers at the state agricultural schools began to announce new advances in poultry science, as it had come to be called. They succeeded in breeding broilers with bloodlines that helped them grow faster to market size and made them meatier when they reached that size. They bred birds whose ability to change grain into meat—their feed conversion ratio—was more and more efficient. The scientists also studied poultry diseases and developed vaccines and antibiotics that made it possible for the chickens to be kept in close quarters, and they helped develop new technologies to make mechanical processing more efficient and easier.

We call an insignificant sum of money "chicken feed," but in fact, chicken feed is what built the modern broiler industry. In the 1950s and 1960s, feed mills bought processing plants—places where previously farmers could sell their birds in small, occasional lots. The new processing plant owners wanted to make the most efficient use of their expensive investments in property, labor, and machinery. So they began to contract with local farmers to raise broilers, and bought the birds at a per-bird price—much as a pieceworker in a factory is paid not by how long he works, but by how many pieces he completes.

Now companies that traditionally manufactured food for livestock and pets—companies like Ralston Purina, Cargill, Inc., Tyson, and Wayne Feeds—also began to be in the business of producing chicken for the American table. And in this "vertical integration"—complete ownership from feed to chick to finished marketable product—the feed companies saw a tremendous opportunity for profit. Anyone can scoop up some of that money. A stockbroker for the investment counseling firm of A. G. Edwards chose Tyson Foods stock as his "best bet" for the week back in early spring 1994. The Springdale, Arkansas–based company "announced a major expansion of its chicken production capacity with the following results," he wrote. "Foodservice share should increase; increasing consumer demand for the company's products can be satisfied. These developments, together with Tyson's strong financial position and improving cost control, should make Tyson attractive for conservative investors at prices below $26 a share."

But conventional genetics have carried the chicken just about as far as it can go. Now poultry science researchers work to create chickens with genetic material from other species, seeking to make chickens that can be kept in ever-closer confinement, that are less vulnerable to stress and disease.

Perhaps, say the scientists, they will eventually be able to change even the way chickens look—perhaps they'll even be able to develop a chicken like that wistful poultryman wanted, the top-profit bird with four breasts and no legs. Certainly it should be possible for scientists to use genetic engineering to develop a chicken with leaner meat and more of it; maybe they can come up with a way to get more white meat and less dark from a chicken. Maybe the poultry bioengineers can use the same technology that aquaculture bioengineers are working on now, a way to "grow" fish flesh without an actual fish ever being involved.

Dr. Lyman Crittendon, a research geneticist at Michigan State University, has worked with the USDA and succeeded in developing a chicken with a genetic "vaccination" against viruses. He's done this by incorporating genetic material from the viruses themselves in the chicken's own DNA.

Another poultry researcher, Ruth Shuman, a former faculty member at North Carolina State University who is now president of a bioengineering company in Minneapolis, has concentrated mostly on disease resistance. "Avian influenza wipes out whole poultry houses," she says, "and salmonella is always present in poultry producers' minds, so genetic resistance would be helpful. While they have rigorous testing programs for this on the farm, this would save everyone time and money."

Moreover, says Shuman, scientists hope to locate the genes in chicken that control the way birds gain weight; doing so would make it possible to manipulate the chickens' DNA to make them produce more meat and less body fat.

Consumers would benefit, she says, because they would get precisely the kind of chicken they want: lean, tender, meaty, and cheap. Besides, she adds, "I'm not sure that birds have preferences about their body shapes. If it's not compatible with thriving (that is, if the changes don't make the birds healthier), it's not compatible for productivity. So if it's good for the chicken, it's good for the industry."

And these changes would, of course, be very good for the industry—at least the industry leaders like Tyson. Because poultry companies like Tyson could own the patent for such genetically engineered chickens, the companies would then truly "own" chickens from top to bottom. And no one could raise such chickens without paying the companies for the privilege.

Most of the country's broiler-raising farmers are in the Deep South, where the processing plants relocated to avoid the need for high-priced union labor. Processing plants in the North and West were abandoned or closed, leaving former employees jobless and farmers who wanted to grow chickens without anywhere to sell them. (Jim's employees are unionized, a fact that he acknowledges makes his company unusual—even as it may disprove the assertion that affordable chicken can be processed only in nonunion plants.) As a result the work force in contemporary chicken plants is almost completely composed of minority women, usually African-American women, who spend their days on their feet in cold, wet packing houses. Today an average of ninety chickens pass by a packing house worker every minute, up from the sixty birds she had to handle every minute in the 1980s. Those high speeds, combined with the repetitiveness of the small task each worker must do as the birds pass along the packing lines, contribute to high rates of carpal tunnel syndrome and other physical stress–related ailments. But since most of the poultry processing workers in this country are not offered health insurance, the injuries often go untreated, and eventually the worker loses the only income she has.

For the farmer himself there are different but equally onerous costs. The poultry company and the farmer sign a short-term contract, usually for about three months, and the poultry company provides everything the farmer needs to raise the chicks to market size. A processing company's truck delivers the chicks and the feed; the processor pays for veterinary care as the birds grow. Another company truck picks up the grown birds, and very often the company pays to have the sheds cleaned before the next shipment of chicks arrives.

The farmer, meanwhile, has likely mortgaged the house and/or the farm to build the very specialized sheds, which typically cost about $100,000 each. To keep transportation costs low, processors usually prefer that growers have more than one shed. So the farmer assumes the risk of the long-term debt, while the processor benefits from the safety of a short-term contract. And if for any reason the farmer decides later that chicken-rearing is not for him—or if he is not offered new contracts every three months—he is left with those specialized and expensive sheds, which are difficult to convert to other uses. Processors often offer premiums to farmers who have low death rates and whose flocks use feed most efficiently, so it is in the farmer's interest to watch his flocks carefully.

Jim hedges his bets as a processor in a small way: he is also a broiler grower in the complex kind of legal corporate organization that lets him sell the birds he raises to his own company. Park Farms buys from other growers as well, but it is Jim's farms that we will tour on this soft spring day.

We start at an inconspicuous low building in a light-industry area inside the Canton city limits. No sign hints at its occupant; it looks like an insurance office or a shipping concern or any of a number of small local businesses.

The first clue that this is no office building lies just inside the door: instead of a welcome mat, a shallow tray filled with a clear solution requires anyone who enters to step through it. It's a foot wash, and its purpose is to protect the vulnerable chicks from the bacteria in the outside world. This is Park Farms' hatchery, and to tour it I must don some heavy, disinfected rubber galoshes.

The hatchery is under the supervision of Indian-born Sabu Kuruvilla, a slight, courtly forty-year-old who's been with the company for about five years. Besides the millions of chicks incubated here, Sabu also oversees the fourteen employees, who rotate job duties as each cycle of egg-hatching proceeds. Sabu expects to double production shortly, he says, which will create four more full-time jobs.

The eggs themselves come from a farm called Peterson Arbor Acres in Gainesville, Georgia; they are a White Plymouth cross, chosen because these birds grow fast and have good feed efficiency, Sabu says. Park Farms does not own the farm whose hens lay these eggs, nor does it own the company that manufactures feed for the growers; in that respect, Park Farms is not totally integrated. But these eggs are from chickens whose sole use is laying eggs to grow into broilers; although you could eat them for breakfast, Sabu says, you probably wouldn't, simply because they would never make it to your supermarket.

The boxes of eggs, 360 to a cardboard crate, arrive at the hatchery every week. They are protected within their boxes, nestled in cardboard flats of 45 eggs each. Sabu says the company hatches 212,400 eggs a week.

The eggs have definite climatic needs from the moment they arrive at the hatchery. They arrive at a temperature of about sixty-five degrees and a relative humidity of about seventy percent. Soon after their arrival they are slowly warmed to around ninety-nine degrees in eighty-five percent humidity, where they will stay until they hatch. Employees load the cardboard flats onto trolleys that hold five thousand eggs each; these trolleys are designed to fit snugly and efficiently into the Chick-Master setters—machines that do for these eggs what hens used to do.

The eggs spend eighteen days in one of the eight Chick-Master machines, which are designed to slowly, gently tilt and retilt the eggs so the developing embryos won't be damaged. Setting hens do this instinctively, turning the eggs with their beaks in a gentle periodic nudging. Each setting room has a capacity of ninety-three thousand eggs, Sabu says, and my head begins to whirl from these massive numbers. Naturally, power supplies are critical to keep the machines doing what they are meant to do. The hatchery keeps a backup generator on-line at all times, to take over if the power is disrupted for any reason.

On the eighteenth day the eggs are moved from the Chick-Masters to the hatching room. The trolleys are designed to slide snugly into these darkened, temperature- and humidity-controlled "closets." It will be two to three days before all the chicks are hatched; Sabu says the hatching rate is about eighty-five percent. There is no way to know until the eggs hatch how many are male and how many are female, although it doesn't really matter. Both sexes will be raised to market size, he tells me, because the birds will be killed before they are old enough to become sexually active.

The hatching room is the first area that begins to smell like chickens: it has a definite, not unpleasant, eggy smell, the scent of raw yolks. That's logical, actually, since the chicks survive on the nutrition they draw from the yolks for the first several days of their lives after hatching. Eggshells and small bits of fluffy feathers litter the racks.

From the hatching room the chicks are moved by trolley to the vaccinating room. Their peep-peep-peeping is shrill, and they are as charming as any chick in a child's book. Two employees casually but quickly grab the chicks from their trolley trays, sending them down a slightly inclined chute that will carry them in a circle on a conveyor belt past the women vaccinators. Deftly and quickly, the women pluck up chicks, holding them against a machine that injects the baby birds with a vaccine against Marek's disease, an ailment that causes cancerous tumors in chickens. The vaccine is dyed green so the women can see that the chick has been properly injected: it makes a brief slight stain on the birds' yellow fluff.

Each vaccination station—there are five—has an automatic click-counter, and the women drop the vaccinated chicks in open, deep-sided plastic trays until they reach a certain number, usually a hundred. Then a new box is begun. The filled boxes of chicks are sent through a machine that mists them with a combination of antibiotics and vaccines against two other viruses. Then, at last, the boxes of peeping chicks are stacked one atop the next until they can be loaded onto trucks.

We are riding in Jim's pickup truck, a newish model with every comfort, including a car phone. We are on our way to see one of Park Farms' seven grow-out operations, rolling through the gentle countryside that Jim has seen his whole life. The countryside is largely rural, but there are few active farms left. Instead, there are mostly fairly new houses, set far back from the road in several-acre plots used to grow huge expanses of lawn. This land is more valuable when developers can split it up and sell as these mini-estates than it is when it is used for farming.

Jim is an attractive man in a raw-boned way; he is tanned and fit, and his graying hair curls at the back of his collar. His manner is forthright and blunt; he is obviously shrewd and often kind. He wears a polo shirt and khakis, little jewelry; he displays his affluence in the discreet cut of his clothes. He is telling me that everything in the poultry industry conspires against a smallhold farmer and that much of the reason for that lies at the feet of the American shopper. "They want cheap chicken," he says, "and this is the only way they can get it. The system only works if a grower can get volume and efficiency. Our packing plant can't accommodate someone who's only interested in raising a handful of birds; the machinery is expensive and so is the labor, and I've got to have it running all the time to make it profitable."

Moreover, he says, a maze of government regulations concerning workplace safety, cleanliness, and labor relations makes it impossible for a small processor to make a go of it. If he killed ten birds a day, he'd be held to the same standards as a processor who kills ten thousand birds a day—and maintaining those standards is expensive. He has to have volume enough to cover those costs.

So volume is what he demands—and gets—from the seven growers, including himself, who raise chickens for Park Farms. Each farm has ten chicken houses on twenty to twenty-five acres, which means each farm raises about 170,000 birds every six weeks. The grower gets the seventh week off while Park Farms' employees clean the sheds and, once or twice a year, bulldoze out the layers of packed feathers, excrement, and bedding sawdust that the birds are raised on. This material is valuable fertilizer, says Jim; on his own farms, the ones we're visiting today, he composts it and uses it to nourish the grain crops his farm managers grow to feed the birds. Other Park Farms' growers get their chickens' feed from the company.

The sheds are equipped with heating systems and large fans to keep the birds at optimal comfort. Cool or cold weather is less of a problem to a chicken grower—the buildings can always be heated if the removable sides are in place—than hot weather. In hot, high-humidity seasons, the birds cannot cool themselves in the crowded sheds, and even the fans can bring little relief. In those circumstances the birds may die in staggering numbers. It is among the risks that chicken growers in the South, where hot weather lasts from February to November, must assume.

The six weeks that the farmer invests in his flocks are busy ones. He must constantly monitor food and water availability and make sure that the temperatures in the shed are at their best for the birds. He may work day and night for those six weeks, although it is unlikely that he will work all day and all night for the entire time. The chickens are immediately vulnerable if the power goes off at the farm, say, for example, in a thunderstorm; the automatic waterers and feeders stop working without electricity, and so does the heating-and-cooling machinery.

At first the farmer feeds the young chick a low-calorie blend of grains to help it mature without outgrowing its heart or its legs. It took chicken farmers and scientists a little while to understand that those are real problems for these specially bred birds. But eventually they realized that it is possible to overfeed a carefully bred chick—one with a very high feed efficiency rating—and so cause it to rupture its own heart or grow so fast that its legs cannot support its weight.

Jake Ramey is a farm manager for one of Jim's farms. He reckons that he'll lose about five percent of the chickens he takes delivery on, birds that will die because they can't compete for food or water, or because they are runts, or from heart attacks. Park Farms picks up dead birds every day and sells them to a rendering plant, explains Ramey; the money from that sale goes to Park Farms, not to the grower.

When the Park Farms truck comes to pick up the fully grown chickens, they'll weigh about 4.5 pounds each, but each bird will lose some .75 pound in processing, he says. This is, he thinks, a good return.

And Jim Pastore, broiler grower, will get paid by Jim Pastore, Park Farms owner, for every bird that passes USDA inspection in the packing plant.

Jake Ramey takes home a paycheck just like a factory employee.

We stop for lunch at a small café that Jim says is known for its excellent hamburgers. I take the hint and order one, and am amused when his order of "the usual" is delivered: a grilled chicken sandwich, no mayonnaise, on a whole wheat bun. Several people greet Jim by name as we settle in to eat our lunches.

We talk about bacterial contamination in raw chicken and in eggs, and for the first time I see Jim's tough side. The salmonella problem in raw chicken is only on the flesh, not deep within the meat, he says. Consumers should not worry about it if they take care in preparing and in cooking, seeing that they keep work surfaces clean and cook the birds thoroughly. If consumers knew how to deal with raw poultry, there would be no salmonella problem at all in chicken, he says; it makes a strong argument for irradiation, the practice of bombarding foodstuffs with low doses of radiation to destroy harmful bacteria.

But wait, I say. Why should the people who buy these chickens even have to worry whether their food is clean and safe and wholesome? Is it possible that our present system of rearing chickens—the close confinement, the high-speed mechanized packing lines—exacerbates the problem of bacterial contamination? What might happen if we reconsidered our methods of poultry production, if we attacked salmonella as a symptom of a larger problem, rather than as a problem in its own right?

"Young lady," Jim says, gently but firmly, "I admire your drive and your quest. But no one can change this system. It's too late. We can't go backwards. The consumer wants cheap food, and this is how it gets produced."

A poultry packing house is no place for the squeamish. The millions of Americans who casually, cheerfully eat chicken five to seven times a week apparently don't stop to consider that the chicken came from a once-living bird. They want to eat the flesh, but they don't want to acknowledge its cost. As a result, shocking exposés like the mid-1980s *60 Minutes* episode on salmonella contamination in poultry processing plants play to a nation of horrified viewers—people who have lost the understanding that their hunger for lean meat can only be satisfied by the butchering of billions of birds.

I am not squeamish as Park Farms' chief executive officer, Ted Hawk, prepares to lead me on the tour, although he is afraid that I will be. "Are you sure you want to see the actual killing?" he asks over and over before we begin. Yes, I assure him, it won't make me queasy. At home, I tell him, I buy my chicken at the kind of old-fashioned poultry shop that Jim says can't survive, the kind where the birds you choose are killed and dressed before your eyes. Someone has to kill all these birds, I say, if we Americans are to have the cheap, constant chicken we seem to demand.

The birds arrive at the factory in crates on flatbed trucks, some six thousand birds at a time. They don't spend much time on the back of the trucks waiting to be processed because these specialized birds don't have much tolerance for stress. It's important to Park Farms to get them into the processing rooms as quickly as possible, to prevent as much loss by sudden death as possible.

A man picks up the crates and tips them through a chute that deposits the noisy, confused birds on a conveyor belt. The belt moves very slowly, but it moves, and its movement puts the birds off guard. A surprised chicken doesn't run, it squats; that is what these birds do in reaction to the moving floor.

Inch by inch they are shunted into a darkened room. The darkness calms the birds, Hawk tells me, or at least it makes them wary enough to quiet themselves. In this darkened room, lit only by the kind of red lamps that one sees in photographic darkrooms—a kind of light that chickens, apparently, can't see—a couple of employees grab the chickens, one by one, and hang them upside down, by the feet, on a moving line about ten feet off the ground. A chicken with its feet in the air is, again, a sort of astonished chicken, says Hawk; when you see pictures of women carrying live chickens in foreign marketplaces, the birds are held upside down because it makes them easier to handle.

It is at this moment, for me, when the chickens seem to stop being living things and become simply a commodity. The line of silent, hanging chickens moves along slowly, inexorably, toward the next room, and it is almost impossible to fathom so many chickens going to their deaths. From this moment on, they could be car parts or any other kind of component in an assembly-line plant.

Of course, there is the small matter of killing them.

As the birds are moved along the line, they emerge into another darkened room. As the line carries the birds forward, their breasts brush against a metal plate; Hawk says the con-

tact soothes the disoriented birds and quiets them even further. Eventually, the metal plate is replaced with a device
that administers a low-level electrical shock to the chickens.
The shock stuns but does not kill them. They are, however,
not conscious when they reach the next step. Or at least they
are not supposed to be conscious.

Now the carefully designed machinery catches the birds'
heads, holding them snugly so that a spinning, cunningly
sharp blade can slit the chickens' throats. It is important,
says Hawk, that the adjustments be precise: the blade should
cut the birds' jugulars but should not sever the heads or
the spinal cord, because the birds will not bleed freely
and properly if they are dead through the next few feet of
the line.

The line propels the birds over catch basins that are gory
with crimson blood, and it is along the next ten feet or so of
machinery that the birds expire, bled to death. It is one man's
job to watch the birds go by, using his hands and a knife to
catch any birds that the machine may have missed. The job is
psychologically exhausting, Hawk says, and employees who
have this job are rotated frequently into other jobs to relieve
them of the stress.

I watch this aspect of the process for a few silent minutes. It appears that the birds, already stunned, do not suffer
unduly, and Hawk has convinced me that every step possible
is taken so that this is true. Like his boss, Ted Hawk seems
an honorable man and a nice one; his open, bluff face encourages friendly feelings. Still, I wish every person who
blandly orders a McChicken sandwich had to come face-to-
face, just once, with this small killing room. We should know
the cost of our appetites, I think.

The next steps along the line carry the now-dead chickens through a vat of soapy water to wash away the dust and
grime from their feathers, and through a pair of automated

plucking machines. The pluckers use rubber "fingers" to brush the wet feathers from the birds; the first is fairly gentle and removes the larger feathers, the second, rougher, gets almost all the pin feathers. In the process sometimes the dead birds' heads pop off; dozens of them litter the concrete floor and gutters.

Now the birds, still hanging by their feet, are carried into the next room, where a clever bit of machinery sorts them into dual lines. Here, on elevated platforms, employees—mostly women—act as backups to the mechanical eviscerators that remove the chickens' guts, lop off any remaining heads, and generally render them into the condition we find them at the supermarket. Two USDA inspectors, both men, work here, too: every chicken goes by one or the other, and every bird gets its own personal split-second inspection.

The birds are graded by size—Hawk tells me that the plant packs different sizes on different days—and many of the birds continue to the last step in processing, where they are cut up, or the breasts are removed for skinning and boning and trimming into quick-cooking nuggets. Most of this chicken will be packed under Park Farms' own label, although some, by contract arrangement, will carry store brands that do not indicate where the chicken came from.

Everything in the cavernous, cool packing rooms is wet and as clean as could reasonably be expected. The employees move about briskly, but they look happy enough. I have seen no evidence of mistreatment of bird or person. I have, in fact, seen a great deal of concern about humane treatment both for the employees and for the chickens that come into this factory as living things and leave it as "product."

It is a model of efficiency, this processing plant.

■   ■   ■

Park Farms has made Jim a prosperous man. He wants to show me the house and barn that he is building, a place that will be open to schoolchildren as a sort of living museum where they can see how a working farm operates.

We see the barn first as we drive up the rutted dirt road: it is an extraordinary thing, the kind of barn that no one can afford to build anymore, the kind that is falling to rack and ruin all across the country. Its high-hipped roof is capped with a weather vane; copper sheathing gilds the arches over doors and trim.

On this farm, Jim says, he will keep cows, sheep, chickens, and goats so the children can see them. No horses—he confesses that he is afraid of horses—and no pigs because pigs smell. But the children who visit will be able to see a cow milked and be able to pet sheep and goats.

He thinks that he will offer schoolchildren the opportunity to grow small plots of cash crops. The children "will harvest what they've grown, and they can keep the profits." It would be a good school project, he says.

Jim shares my concerns about the way agriculture is headed in this country, and he maintains that all this is the proof of it. He wants to create a place where children can gain a sense of how food is produced, even though no real food will be produced here, except as a sort of curiosity. But it is important, he says. We have to do something to help our children maintain their connection to the land.

A stone's throw from the nearly completed barn is another huge building. What's that going to be, I say, knowing but teasing. Will that be the visitors' center? No, yelps Jim, an unlikely blush springing to his cheeks: that is his house. It's been under construction for almost two years and won't be finished for yet another.

Eventually, Jim will move into this lovely mansion on the hill, set far back from all the roads around it, protected and private. He will live in this house and run a pretend farm, a well-meant if impotent farm of fantasy.

And so it may be that the last farm in Jim Pastore's birthplace will end up as an agricultural theme park.

# Building a Better Bird

*I*f there is a hard way to do a thing, says David Wilson, he will find it. That's just the way he is. He didn't even get born the easy way: when the doctor showed up to attend his mother, the infant David had arrived, unassisted.

And that is why, he goes on to say, he set about figuring out a way to change the way chicken is produced in this country, albeit on a very small scale.

David is a native Kentuckian who still farms a little. "Not as much as I should do, though," he says. "I need to get some dirt in my hands." He's not able to do as much farming as he'd like these days, however, because he's spending an awful lot of time on the road. He describes himself as "the dog-and-pony-show man" for Wilson Fields, headquartered in Louisville, Kentucky, probably the smallest poultry company in the United States. David lent his name to the company when it was founded in 1988; investors, taken with his ideas, put up the capital.

But David was not raised as a farmer. His childhood was "near idyllic," he says, and the family was prosperous enough to school him in private academies where he boarded during the school year. He farms by choice, not because it is the only thing he knows how to do.

It was while David was raising squab—young pigeons—for the white-tablecloth restaurant trade that he became friends with some very fine chefs. Those chefs, he recalls, kept telling him about the superb chickens they had tasted in Europe, specifically in France. Maybe, thought David, we ought to figure out a way to raise chickens like that here.

So he booked himself a trip to France. There he met poultry growers who carefully shepherded flocks of birds bred from bloodlines going back seven hundred years or more, the stock viewed by the French government as a national treasure. The chickens in France, he learned, were encouraged to "free range," or to take themselves out into the yards outside their barns. Because they were raised in smaller flocks than those in typical American poultry houses, the birds endured less stress, so they didn't need antibiotics in their food and water to keep diseases away. Fed only grain, rather than feed that included the ground-up feathers and carcasses of other chickens, these birds didn't fight with each other and showed no signs of the cannibalism that is among the banes of the American poultry industry. And because these birds were raised almost three weeks longer than their American counterparts, their flesh had a succulence and deep flavor that is rarely found in chicken anymore.

David Wilson, hardheaded and intelligent, began to think.

■    ■    ■

At 50, David is a strapping man, lean through the legs and hips but endowed with a modest burgher's belly. His graying hair is carelessly barbered, and his fingernails are trimmed close to the quick. He wears T-shirts and blue jeans and high-topped lace-up leather farmers' work boots as he makes his way through the world, using a spraddle-legged bouncing-on-the-balls-of-his-feet gait to get where he's going. He is shrewd enough to see that there are some advantages in being underestimated.

I have come to Kentucky to see Wilson Fields' free-range, antibiotic-free specially bred chickens, both in the growing houses and in the packing plant. It has fallen to David to tend to me, David the dog-and-pony-show man.

It is high summer on this visit, the hilly countryside in Adair County rich with the deepening blue-green that comes as summer relaxes into its last lushness. In the distance the hills melt into a softening haze that gentles the horizon. It is a kind of countryside that is easy for many of us to forget exists: smallhold farm after smallhold farm, twisting narrow country lanes leading from one to another, and almost all the farms with a half-acre patch of tobacco. David-the-farmer looks at each farm, each patch of tobacco, intently, knowingly, as they roll by one after another; he points out whose crop looks good and whose looks poorly. And he observes that no matter how good the crops look, tobacco is a commodity with a very limited future. These Kentucky farmers, he says, will need something to replace it.

Before World War II, David explains, lots of Kentucky farmers raised chickens as part of a larger cycle of farm life. They sold those chickens to local processing plants, who in turn sold them to people who lived in the neighborhood, in a manner of speaking. But after the war all the little processors got bought up and shut down, and Kentuckians stopped growing chickens on land that often is too hilly to be good for much else. The poultry industry moved farther south or to the Delmarva peninsula, land shared by Delaware, Maryland, and Virginia.

When David returned from that trip to France, he brought with him the exclusive rights to American use of a special line of chicken-breeding stock. The breed is called *Label Rouge* in France, red being the mark of excellence there, as a blue ribbon is in this country. But having the rights to the breeding stock was just the tiniest part of the picture.

Eventually, through a combination of serendipity and sweat, David found a poultry house in Quebec, Canada, where the young chicks could be quarantined for a month before they would be allowed into the United States. Once the birds were released from quarantine, they were dispatched to an Arkansas brooder, who cared for the birds as they began to lay their special, valuable eggs. The eggs were sent on to a Missouri hatchery where they could be nurtured into the second generation of chicks, chicks that would be raised in special ways for the table. The chicks are shipped to Wilson Fields' growers, most of them in Kentucky and North Carolina.

Culinary quality is David's benchmark, and he believes that a chicken raised in a way that lets the chicken be a chicken will give it a flavor that can't be bested.

Ease of production, volume, efficiency, packing house speeds—all those things are barely even secondary to David. The first thing that counts is whether this chicken tastes good.

And David's chickens do taste good—spectacularly good, in fact. But I get ahead of myself.

Leon and Laverne Kessler have raised chickens for upward of thirty years, but they had never raised chickens the way David has had them do.

It is crushingly hot when we arrive unannounced at the Kesslers' farm on Fry Ridge Road near Columbia. David assures me that our surprise visit will not discomfort the Kesslers, that they'll be glad to see him—and thus me.

He pulls the car up near the poultry house, parks it, and wipes his brow in almost one motion. It is the Kesslers' adult daughter, Betty Simpson, who sees us first, and David hails her, shouting down the long yard. He draws himself up to wait for her alongside the Kesslers' organic garden, and she makes her way up the gentle hill in the sort of hurried leisure that indicates she's eager to talk to David but that it's too hot to rush.

Once we've all been introduced, David leaves us to wade into the garden. He plucks green beans—a couple—from their bushes and passes one along to me. They are sweet and tender and crisp, and because I know this is an organic garden, I hesitate not even a millisecond before discovering this.

The garden is alive with butterflies; birds dart here and there. A russeted bird perched on a power line breaks into its music, and Betty asks David what kind of bird that is. "A song sparrow, I think," he says. "That's not a meadowlark's song." Laverne has joined us. She points out a bluebird poised nearby, and we all just stand there a moment, the sun beating down on our heads, listening. It is a lovely moment.

We begin to talk about the chickens. Betty ambles into the garden herself, breaks off an ear of corn, shucks it and gives it wordlessly to David, who wordlessly breaks it in half and hands me a piece. "I didn't know if you'd want to eat it raw like that," Betty says, apologetically, but I can't answer: my mouth is busy with that sweet, sun-warmed corn, milky and crisp, the smell of the silk still lingering about the ear.

"We love these chickens," says Laverne. "We just love them. At first, when David talked to us about raising them, we weren't sure. But we love them now. I'd never want to go

back to raising chickens the old way—and we've been growing chickens for thirty years."

The birds in the poultry house are a couple of weeks old,
I'm told. They are fully feathered but a long way from being
fully grown. They'll begin to go outside when they reach their
third week of life. Until then the young chickens need to establish their preferred places in the poultry house, need to
come to see that long, low shed as home.

Stepping into the poultry house, I can see immediately
that these birds, these methods, have little to do with Jim Pastore's. These chickens, deeply feathered, mostly white, scat-
ter before us at first, chirring reassurance to one another, but
they settle quickly and soon are curious enough to walk up to
us and inspect us with shiny eyes, cocking their heads this
way and that to get the best image.

"Hello, you little sillies," says David affectionately to the
chicks. "Hello, all you silly little birds. You're just little silly
things, aren't you?"

To understand how different these birds are from chickens raised in industrial ways, we have to draw some compar-
isons. Their legs are longer, for one thing, because they need
to be strong enough to run and hop and jump around; David
says the thigh bone in one of his chickens will be two inches
long or more, compared to considerably less than that in
an industrial bird. Their heads are bigger, too—"We want
them to have some brains on them," says David, in expla-
nation—and they seem more willing to walk, more confident somehow.

Many of the chickens bred for contemporary poultry
production have a good bit of Cornish blood in their lines,
says David. That produces a quiet bird, a bird that will sit
motionless for hours if permitted. "Those birds," says David,
shaking his head, "those birds won't move if you put a boot
to them." But that is not what David wants in his birds.

We stand sweating in the poultry house for some thirty minutes, watching the birds and talking about the poultry industry in general, these chickens in particular. Laverne tells me that these birds are virtually never sick, that she's never had to administer anything significant in the way of antibiotics to this flock or the ones she's raised for David before. They're healthy, she says, because there are fewer of them in a flock—about seven thousand in this house, compared to the eighteen thousand or more in a conventional house of the same size—and because they get up and move around. In fact, she says, there is a ratio, a formula that's followed for these birds: they get nine times as much room outside, per bird, as they get inside. Naturally, conventionally raised chickens don't have access to the outside at all.

It is only as we step out of the house, back into the bright, hot midday sun, that I realize that we've spent a half hour inside a poultry house—and I didn't notice the smell.

Laverne laughs when I remark on that. "Oh, it's real different than the way we used to do it," she says. "Used to be, you got in there and got out again as fast as you could, because of the ammonia smell. It would make your eyes just water and water."

For dinner that night David cooks two "La Belle Rouge" chickens for four of us, together with a salad and some boiled potatoes tossed with butter. Wilson Fields calls its premium chickens La Belle Rouge—"the beautiful red," in English— because the French government has given its special chickens an *"appellation controlée,"* like Champagne wine. Only chickens raised in France from those bloodlines may be called *Label Rouge.* There's good bread with dinner, and fresh fruit, sliced, for dessert. David works silently to assemble the meal, refusing all offers of help, while I talk with Tim Matz and Doug Gossman, two of Wilson Fields' executives.

The thirty-four-year-old Tim, blond and lean, is carefully barbered and dressed in the casually elegant style that bespeaks a certain affluence. He tells me that he brings marketing, sales, and "entrepreneurial expertise" to Wilson Fields, together with some skills in corporate organization. He struggles to give himself a title when I ask. Finally he says, "Just call me an officer of the company."

Doug, forty-five, is the company's president and has been since November 1993. He, too, is sandy-haired and fit, but his features are blunter than Tim's. He's been in the food business since 1971, and his skills include an understanding of food trends in the restaurant industry, knowledge of the wholesale meat trade, and an appreciation of the public's desires in fine food, he says.

Both men are married; both are the fathers of four-year-old children. Their families live in Louisville, where Wilson Fields is headquartered; they have come to Columbia, where the processing plant is located, to meet me, to talk about their company.

The house, which belongs to a former business associate of Tim's, is spectacularly situated on a bluff with views of Lake Cumberland both east and west. The sun is a red fireball in the western sky, sliding down into the hills as we arrive, and before long, the soft hot night fully surrounds the house. The chittering of insects fills the air, so loud that it outshouts the stereo that Tim turned on as soon as he entered the house; both Tim and Doug refer to the insects as crickets. I know that they are not, in fact, crickets—their song is not the creek-creek that crickets make in rubbing their wings with their legs—but I am not sure what they are. David does not correct Doug and Tim, perhaps because they do not ask him to name the insects making the night music. But when I ask him, he tells me that they are katydids. "Listen," he says, "you can hear them saying their names: Katy did. Katy did."

Tim and Doug are talking about some of the problems that have plagued the small company. Distribution is difficult, says Doug, because all the problems of supply have not yet been worked out, and sometimes there is demand for chicken when the company has no chicken to offer.

The company has eighteen growers in Kentucky, another twenty in North Carolina, Doug says; most growers have one or two poultry houses, raising fewer than fifteen thousand birds every sixty-three to sixty-five days. The company sells chickens to upscale supermarkets and whole-food markets under two labels, which are actually two different bloodlines of chicken, he says. One is called Penny Royal, which David says later was "designed to replace the bastardized, shimsham, industrial bird; it's raised free-range, antibiotic-free." The other is called La Belle Rouge, the same breed of bird we saw at the Kesslers' that morning. Most markets carry one or the other, but few carry both, Doug says. Through distributors around the country, the company also sells to the restaurant trade. Eventually, says Tim, Penny Royal will be the company's retail label; La Belle Rouge will be reserved for the white-tablecloth restaurant trade and the very finest gourmet supermarkets. "It's the difference between a Mercedes, a Cadillac, and a Chevy," he says, the Chevy being, of course, a conventionally produced American chicken.

Both birds average about three and a half pounds, dressed, says Doug, and both will retail for $1.99 to $2.99 a pound, that dollar's difference being the retailer's latitude for markup. Male birds will weigh a little more; female birds will weigh a little less. Wilson Fields sells their whole birds without giblets, a move that David instigated because the delicate organ meats tucked in the cavity spoil quickly.

Virtually all Wilson Fields chickens are sold fresh, Doug says, although a few customers—perhaps five percent—

prefer to buy the birds frozen, in the name of longer shelf life for their clientele. But because of differences in the processing plant, Doug says—differences I'll see myself the next day— a customer would be hard-pressed to tell the difference between a frozen-and-thawed Wilson Fields bird and a fresh one.

But some of the problems of supply are being resolved, says Doug. Soon, Wilson Fields should be hatching its own chicks, and the company has designs for larger poultry sheds that will allow growers to grow four times the chickens they are now able to. The houses will be divided into four separate flocks, which will give the chickens the idea that they are in small flocks; that was David's idea, Doug points out. "David says sometimes you have to think like a chicken," says Doug, laughing at what he clearly believes to be David's inexplicable mind.

Tim will tell me later that Wilson Fields is built on what David has dubbed "the four fors": for the welfare of the farmer, for the welfare of the environment, for the welfare of the chickens, and for the welfare of the consumer. "If we practice those, we should accomplish our mission," Tim will tell me, pointing out that the company has very carefully designed water-treatment systems for the water used in processing, and that the company packs its birds in biodegradable packing materials.

Dinner is ready. I cannot help admiring the two plump birds David has roasted after rubbing them with olive oil and lemon juice and garlic. They are perfectly browned, their skin thin and crisp; their fragrance fills the kitchen, and suddenly I am ravenously hungry. Look, says David, pointing to the cookie sheet he's roasted the birds on. Look, there's not a half-cup of fat in that pan. He carves the chickens roughly, piles the meat on a platter, and we adjourn to the dinner table.

The business of passing dishes and filling plates fills the first few moments at the table, but soon enough we are all served. I cannot resist tearing off a shred of chicken and popping it into my mouth, and I am instantly rewarded. Here is a chicken that simply tastes like chicken. Its meat is tender and moist, with a satisfying succulence. For me the standard for roast chicken was set more than fifteen years ago at a three-table bistro in Tangier, Morocco, the first time I ate a chicken that tasted like a chicken. No chicken I've purchased and cooked myself—no bird I've eaten in any restaurant—since then has ever approached that one.

Tonight, I am thinking, I may have to reset my standard. This is one hell of a chicken.


Without Louise Brown, there might not be genetically engineered animals. From the moment of Brown's birth in 1978 in England, she was famous: she was the first test-tube baby.

The catchy headline phrase notwithstanding, Brown might be more accurately termed the world's first petri dish baby. That's where she was conceived, using an egg from her mother and sperm from her father, by Dr. Stephen Steptoe and Cambridge University physiologist Robert Edwards. Steptoe implanted the fertilized egg in Mrs. Brown's womb, and nine months later, by cesarean section, history was made.

Mrs. Brown wasn't able to conceive by normal means because her fallopian tubes were blocked. That the thirty-one-year-old housewife could deliver a normal, healthy child gave hope to thousands of couples struggling with infertility.

A Louis Harris and Associates survey of some fifteen hundred American women, conducted two months after Louise Brown's birth, showed that 85 percent thought the test-tube method of conception "should be made available to married couples unable to have children," a United Press International story reported at the time. "This widespread sympathy for couples unable to have children may stem partially from the surprising number of women experiencing difficulty conceiving," said *Parents* magazine, which commissioned the poll.

The technology and science that made Louise Brown's birth possible are routine now. Ten years after she was born, an estimated ten thousand children around the world had been conceived in vitro, or "in glass." By the time Brown turns twenty in 1998, she may be the eldest in a family of many thousands more in vitro siblings.

The agricultural scientists who work with livestock knew that the same technologies and science could be put to work to improve the bloodlines and delivery rates of cows, pigs, goats, sheep, and other mammals.

By removing eggs from the donor mother and fertilizing them in vitro, scientists gained the ability to manipulate the genetic structure of the embryos before they were fully formed. The embryos could then be reimplanted, either in another mother or back into the donor's womb.

That's how Pig No. 6707 was created at the USDA's Beltsville, Maryland, laboratories. That's how scientists created a hybrid creature that is half goat and half sheep— the "geep."

Poultry bioengineering is more complicated. Chickens have large eggs, especially as compared with mammals' eggs, and the eggs are enclosed in that hard shell. To work on a chicken embryo, scientists have had to figure out a way to work on an embryo that is inside an egg—inside a chicken. Moreover, a chicken lays only a single egg at a time; scientists couldn't work on many eggs at once, as they can with mammals like pigs that bear large litters.

As a result, bioengineering research on poultry lags behind that work being done on other livestock. But scientists hope they'll be able to make the process more efficient soon.

They believe they'll be able to create new kinds of chickens that grow faster, have leaner meat, need less feed, and have superior disease resistance.

David Wilson's chickens don't grow fast. Their meat is a little leaner than that of conventional chickens, because they move around more. They need more feed, not less, because they grow longer. Their disease resistance is high, but that's because they're raised with lots of space, fresh air, and good feed.

And as I said, David's chickens make fabulous eating. I have found no references, anywhere, to scientists working to develop chickens that taste better.

It is daylight, just, but the sun is not yet risen when David and I meet the next morning. Although the air is cool, the morning's hazy beginnings bode for another steamy, sticky day.

We are going out to visit two other Wilson Fields poultry growers' flocks to see the birds ranging out of their sheds and into their yards. This the birds do two or three times a day, typically early in the morning—it's just past six a.m. when we pull away from the motel—and in the early evening, when the day's heat begins to dwindle. Sometimes they will come out in the middle of the day if the weather is cool.

Early as it is, this is agricultural country, and so we encounter an occasional car or truck as we wend along those twisting country roads. David greets each oncoming driver with a lazy, casual wave of his left hand: the country wave, acknowledging everyone, even people you don't know, as somebody worth greeting. I have noticed, in my time with him, that he extends that courtesy even further in the kind of commonplace meetings that we all have each day. He speaks to the toll-taker on the highway and remarks favorably to the waitress about the caliber of the pie she made for dessert in a little diner. He talks tobacco-growing with the desk clerk at the motel, and he how-dos the strangers we meet in the breakfast room there.

As we ride along, David-the-farmer again eyes the landscape, brightening now as the sun rises, the haze beginning to shimmer in the warming air. He laughs when I tell him that I have learned how to tell time by the plotting of sitcoms on the television, and that is why I no longer wear a watch, since televisions are now easier to find in public places than clocks are. He laughs again when I tell him that this is not a skill I prize very highly, since it bespeaks far too much time in front of the television. He tells time in a different way, he says. We are already heading toward fall, and the signs are threefold: the young birds are off the nests now, feeding and growing and strengthening for the winter; the seed heads on the grasses have begun to dry and turn brown; and the oak trees are done with the growing they will do this season. Those three signs, he says, will lead us into autumn.

David has learned that each week of the year has some plant or flower that is its marker: chicory blooms here along about the first week of July, and then comes Queen Anne's lace. There's something like that for every week of the year, he says, no matter where you live; you just have to take the time to find it and recognize it.

By now we have reached the first of the two farms we'll visit this morning. The people who live here are still abed or are settling in over their breakfasts; we do not see them in the thirty minutes or more we spend looking at the chickens.

It's easy to watch the birds for that long or longer because what chickens do is interesting to watch—and so foreign to most of us, who could live out our entire lives without ever having the opportunity to watch chickens being chickens. The birds are enclosed in a large grassy area, perhaps a quarter of an acre or more; they may go into the house or come into the yard as they wish. Some of these birds, at seven weeks old, jump up in the air, flapping their wings, just for the exercise of it, David says. Sometimes a chicken will rush up to another bird and the two will stare at each other, beak-to-beak, in a chicken dominance game that settles or re-asserts the pecking order. All the birds walk about, pecking at the green shoots of grass, at gravel, at bugs if they can find them. The flock is quiet, except for the sort of throaty mur-muring that forms the birds' conversation with their flock mates. The birds do not, however, peck at each other; neither do they bully one another in any way. With lots of room to get out of each other's way, there is no need for any of that.

At the next farm the scene is very similar. In these pens the chickens perch on tree limbs or on old and rusted equip-ment that rests within the fencing. The birds are curious about us, briefly, and then they go back to the business of be-ing chickens.

David tells me that he has seen a very substantial differ-ence in the kinds of things American farmers have bred into their livestock and the kinds of things that Europeans have bred into theirs. Here, he says, aggressiveness is almost val-ued, and he illustrates that idea with the story of a farmer he knew whose prize bull was so vicious that it eventually put the man in the hospital: "It waited until one day when it could get between the farmer and the gate, and it stove in his ribs, broke just about every bone in his body. But it was a big bull, and that was what the farmer wanted." By contrast, he has seen dairy and beef bulls in Europe so gentle that small children play around their feet and can lead the great beasts by a single rope.

It's the same with chickens, he says. In America we've bred the birds to be big and meaty, and with that comes ag-gressiveness. That's not what he wanted. He wanted birds that could live peacefully with each other, that had the brains to solve their own chicken problems. Having the right blood-lines is a big part of the way to make a chicken cook right and well for the table, says David; giving it the right conditions to grow in is another big part.

There is peace here, a rightness to the picture, that suffuses me with a very quiet joy. The air is sweet and fresh, the day coming on hot; but here, in this spot, there is a timelessness that is the mother of an enduring satisfaction.

As much as I enjoyed my time with Jim Pastore, I did not have these feelings on his farms.

Wilson Fields' processing plant started out years ago as a beef processing plant. It was built in a complicated financing deal that involved some federal money, David says, but when the federal boys came down to see what their money had done, there wasn't any money left. Soon afterward the original owners went to jail. So the new plant stood empty for some 10 of the 12 years it's been on this property.

Converting the plant to poultry processing has not been easy, David says. The rooms aren't the right sizes for the things they're needed for, and the company is already outgrowing this building. A new processing plant is high on the company's wish list.

The chickens are brought to the processing plant in crates of ten birds each, having been caught the night before. Catching these chickens is not especially efficient, says David; the men whose job it is have to run after the birds because these birds are bred for running. Unlike the Cornish-cross stock in conventional poultry houses, these birds don't want to be captured.

It is true that some of the birds are injured in the catching and crating. A few suffer broken wings or legs. It is not something that pleases David, but he thinks that better, bigger crates may help solve the problem.

At the back of the plant, the crates move inside on a wheeled conveyor line. Men reach into the crates and grab chickens, then hang them upside down by the feet on a moving line just as they do at Jim Pastore's plant, or at any other modern poultry processor. Unlike Jim Pastore's birds, however, these birds flutter and struggle; they are not happy about being so helpless, and it shows.

For a time Wilson Fields tried using a very high-tech carbon dioxide stunning machine to make the birds unconscious before the kill. But there were problems with the machine's design, and it didn't do a very good job, so it was reluctantly discarded. It was probably the most humane way to do this to chickens when it worked properly, David says, but when it didn't, it wasn't humane at all.

So now the company has gone back to its original system. The line of birds moves slowly past a man in a blue plastic apron who sits on a folding chair in a screened-in hallway of sorts, open to the outside. As each bird passes the man, he applies a wand with a low direct-current charge to each bird's throat. The birds convulse quickly, briefly, their wings stretching up rigidly toward their tails, and then are still. They are unconscious.

The man who does this job looks relaxed, but he is paying a lot of attention to his work. He is careful to hit each bird correctly on the first try, and he holds the wand at the throat no longer than he must. "There's a lot more going into that than maybe you can see," says David. "He's very good at what he does, very concerned about the birds."

The now-stunned birds continue moving along to the next room, where their throats are slit and they bleed to death. It is hard for those of us who live off the farm to understand, says David, that this is a painless way to die, the birds never regaining consciousness. And the federal government, in the guise of the USDA, agrees that this is absolutely the most humane way to kill chickens.

It is at the next step that one of the key differences in Wilson Fields' processing procedures is evident.

In conventional processing plants the chickens are carried through a very hot—scalding—soapy bath to wash away the dirt from the farm and to soften the follicles that hold the feathers, so as to make plucking easier.

At Wilson Fields a European method is employed. Three stair-stepped tanks of water comprise three separate baths, none of them as hot as conventional processors' single bath. The lower temperatures help preserve the natural oils in the chicken's skin, says David, and that helps keep quality high. Moreover, the birds start in the lowest, dirtiest bath and are moved through progressively cleaner waters, so there is less chance for cross-contamination.

Now the birds are sent through automatic pluckers and on past an employee whose job it is to pull off any remaining pinfeathers, although not many are left on, judging by how she works. Only occasionally does she pluck at a bird, passing most of them along down the line with an inspection rather than an act. David says that's another benefit of the lower-temperature, repeated scaldings over a single, hotter one: the plucking machines can do a better job, even on birds like these with heavy feathering.

Finally, the birds' last step before entering the evisceration room is to have their feet cut off, and their heads, if their heads still remain. A sole employee handles this job, doing both tasks by hand.

It is the first hint that the lines here move far more slowly than they do in an industrial-style plant: both the employee who checks for pinfeathers and the employee who takes off the feet work steadily but easily. The chickens aren't moving past them so quickly that they have to struggle to keep up.

In the next room the chickens are eviscerated by hand, rather than by the machines that conventional processors use. A line of perhaps a dozen employees perform this task, using an elegant scooping motion, fluid and easy, to flip the birds' innards out of their bodies. They wear disposable plastic gloves, and each work station has a foot-operated hot water faucet for them to warm and wash their hands. It is easy to see that there is virtually no damage to the internal organs, and thus little chance of spreading contamination from gut to flesh, one of the ways in which salmonella and other bacterial contaminations are spread. The birds continue past the requisite USDA inspector, who has time to look at each bird for a minute or more.

When at last the birds come off the processing lines, they are sent to the next, highly unusual section of Wilson Fields' processing plant.

Wilson Fields uses an air-chilling method, rather than the water-chilling bath that is the standard in the conventional poultry processing industry. Large stainless-steel racks, on wheels and shaped in a deep V, are fitted with pegs that the chickens rest on. The racks, when loaded, are rolled into a room where the air rushing over them over the span of an hour or two, gradually reduces the birds' temperature to the government standard of 40 degrees or below. USDA guidelines allow this chilling process, whether done by water bath or by cold air, to take as long as sixteen hours, David says; but it is clear to me that that time span is more to accommodate production-line backlogs than to ensure quality. In other words, the processor has 16 hours to get the chickens cooled to that temperature; the government does not suggest that it should take that long to do so, only that it will not tolerate anything longer than that.

Wilson Fields is the only poultry processor in the country, at this writing, that air-chills its chickens. It is unlikely that the poultry industry will rush to follow its lead, however. David's chickens lose two percent of their weight in air chilling. By contrast, federal guidelines allow for a gain of up to ten percent of conventionally produced chickens' weight in water—the gain made in passing chickens through water baths. It's this water, tinted by blood, that shoppers find soaking into the little absorbent squares placed in a tray of cut-up conventional chicken or in the package with a whole fryer. Water is cheap, shrugs David; it's a nice ten-percent profit for the processor. Were every poultry processor in this country to adopt Wilson Fields' air-chilling methods, he says, the accounting books would reflect that combined total of a twelve-percent loss in profits on the first day they switched over.

Most of Wilson Fields' chickens will be sold as whole fryers, but the company is able to process some of them into cut-up fryers, boneless skinless breasts, and the like. Both Doug and Tim told me the night before, over dinner, that they would like the company to do more of that kind of packing—because that's where the profit is, the average American shopper not wishing to invest the time to cut up her own chicken.

Wilson Fields is wooing its fifth flight of investors about the time that I visit. None of the first four flights of investors recouped even a penny, David tells me sadly, wryly. But the company has some promise, and rounding up money is not so difficult. Lots of people, it seems, want to picture themselves becoming Frank Perdue, only in a politically correct way.

I ask David about the direction the company is headed in, building bigger and bigger poultry houses, speeding up processing lines, and increasing capacity. Is that the way he would like to see Wilson Fields go?

He doesn't answer that question directly, being a diffidently self-contained man. Instead, he talks about another idea he's had, one he's beginning to think about rounding up some private philanthropic grant money for.

All these Kentucky farmers, he says, they're going to need something when tobacco isn't a good cash crop for them anymore. They're going to need something to convert to when the government ends tobacco subsidies. But no one is showing these farmers an alternative.

That's what David would like to do. He'd like to buy a tobacco farm as a model and convert it to other uses so other farmers can come visit, study, learn. It wouldn't be a place for the casual public to come and visit, David says, not a showplace for children to visit on school field trips or a theme park. Instead, it would be a working farm, profitable in its own right, that could help farmers lift up their eyes from the soil and see some new ways of thinking.

A farm has to be an integrated system, explains David. It should produce everything that it needs for its operation: the livestock provide organic matter, through their manure, to plow into the soils to enrich and nourish it; the soil grows the feed for the stock; and the farmer can make a dignified, honest living.

"You blow the model, though, the first time you go off the farm to buy tires for the tractor," David says. "And I don't think we're going to convince anyone to go back to farming with mules or horses. Although the Amish do it, very successfully."

I tell David that he sounds like a student of Wendell Berry, another Kentuckian who has gained an impeccable reputation as a farmer, teacher, poet, and essayist, a thoughtful man who has written persuasively and eloquently on our flawed approach to agriculture. David laughs.

"I *am* a student of Wendell Berry's, or I was, way back," he says. "I actually had the nerve to argue with him, back then, although now I realize how dumb I was to do that. I couldn't see what he was saying, couldn't hear it. Berry's hard for me to read, though. He has chosen his words so carefully that you have to take the time to read carefully yourself, to be sure that you understand exactly what he's saying."

I ask David again about the future of Wilson Fields, pressing him a little.

"Dunno," he says finally. "Maybe the answer is that Kentuckians ought to be raising chickens for Kentuckians, and Michigan farmers ought to be raising chickens for Michigan folks. Maybe we ought to be thinking about whether we want cheap food or quality food."

Hardheaded and intelligent, David Wilson is the first person I've met in the poultry industry who even thinks about questions like these.

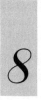

# Two Looks into Two Futures

*W*e've seen how food is grown and produced in this country using two very different approaches, two remarkably different sets of values, and two vastly disparate psychologies. But what does the future portend?

To explore the possibilities, two dedicated proponents for their viewpoints agreed to imagine a future if their methods of food production were adopted.

John C. Sorenson is the general manager for the vegetable division of Asgrow; until 1994 an agricultural supply division of the pharmaceutical company Upjohn, headquartered in Kalamazoo, Michigan. Asgrow has since been sold to a Mexican conglomerate, which is itself a subsidiary of Mexico's largest cigarette manufacturer. John has been with Asgrow for twelve years; he holds a bachelor's degree in biology and chemistry from Defiance College in Defiance, Ohio; credits in postgraduate work from Michigan State University in plant genetics; and a doctorate in biology and genetics from the University of South Carolina. At Asgrow, John is responsible for the development of new varieties of vegetable crops and for the production, sales, and marketing of those varieties.

Asgrow is the largest vegetable seed company in North America. The company is working on dozens of transgenic crops—mostly squashes, cantaloupes, watermelons, cucumbers, lettuce, and tomatoes—in the area of disease resistance, especially viral and fungal resistance. At this writing, Upjohn and Asgrow are awaiting the FDA's approval for a transgenic yellow crookneck squash that includes genetic material from several viruses. The company had hopes that it would be approved in time to make the market in 1995.

John is a burly, affable man who doesn't understand the fuss about bioengineered foods, and particularly doesn't understand the virulent opposition he has encountered from bioengineering's critics. He and the critics of bioengineering are all working toward the same ends: a world in which fewer harmful chemicals are released into the air and water and onto the land; a world in which farmers, already struggling to make a decent living, have a chance to do so with dignity and honor.

John sees the public he serves as threefold: the farmer, of course, but also the men and women who make their living distributing food, and the customer who buys that food for the table. It is the farmer, however, to whom most of Asgrow's research is directed.

"The farmer is, I think, caught in a bind now," says John. "He is in a very difficult situation overall." Most farmers, he says, are keenly aware of their responsibilities concerning the stewardship of the land; they understand the environmental issues that extend beyond their farms. They recognize that the public wants food produced with fewer and fewer toxic agricultural chemicals. But at the same time the farmer must contend with several challenges: to produce a crop as reliably as possible, and as efficiently as possible, for the most profit from the least effort.

"Those things tend to pull in different directions," says John. "So my biggest objective is in developing ways to resolve those tensions. That's why our bioengineering focus is so strongly on disease resistance, as it is with our conventional plant-breeding efforts. Disease resistance helps the farmer be more earth-friendly but not at the expense of reliable production."

To illustrate his point, John paints a vivid picture. A commercial squash grower, who will likely live in the southeastern United States, may plant as much as five times the acreage he needs to make a profit. He does this, John explains, because as much as eighty percent of his crop may be lost to pests and disease. The hidden costs of that overplanting are five times the agricultural chemicals and fertilizers, five times the diesel fuel for the tractor, and five times the seed the farmer actually needs. In addition, says John, that's five times the required acreage devoted to monocrop farming, land that could be used for other crops if squash could be made more reliable. You could argue, he says, that the farmer must work five times harder than he has to—or would have to, if he had access to seeds that had disease or pest resistance bred into them from the start.

John admits that losses as high as eighty percent are not the norm—that's more like twenty percent. But farmers almost always overplant, especially after a bad year. And then the farmer is in a no-win situation, John explains. If the crop comes to harvest in almost its full yield, the farmer loses because prices are lower when there is a lot of his crop at the market. But if he takes a beating due to disease and pests he has less crop to sell, even when prices are good. The deck is stacked, though it's not the farmer who's got the house advantage.

But a field planted with Asgrow's bioengineered, disease-resistant seed would look different, he says. The first thing you'd notice is that it's smaller and that there isn't a spraying rig parked at the side of the field, waiting to be used yet again to spray the vulnerable plants against diseases and pests. "The farmer might look more relaxed," says John, "since he doesn't have to work quite so hard to make his profit."

While the single field of squash that John imagines will still be planted to one crop only, other land on the farm will be available for other crops, he says. In theory, at least, a prudent farmer could spread his risk over several crops, planting less of each one. Asked if he thinks farmers would manage their land in that way, John laughs. "You'd have to talk to the farmers about that, I guess."

According to John, bioengineering does not threaten plant or animal diversity, any more than conventional seed and animal breeding programs do. "We are working now to give plants disease resistance as a way to give them a major share of the market," John says. "You do that because they have superior characteristics to the other similar seeds available. Bioengineering does not change that dynamic."

Moreover, John adds, bioengineering does not threaten diversity of plant breeds through patenting. In fact, he says, the ability to patent plant varieties, granted by Congress in the Plant Variety Patenting Act (PVPA) passed in the early 1970s, encourages research into new varieties. It recognizes that companies who invest large sums of money in research deserve to have that research protected. The PVPA does give a new kind of protection to plant breeders. John says: "We can get utility patents on genes now, which we haven't been able to do with previous breeding because we couldn't characterize and describe the genes' functions before."

In a global sense, soybeans and wheat are often grown from saved seed, "but the ramifications of bioengineering will be more modest than many people who raise that issue believe they will be." He insists that the reason behind patent protection is not to lock the seed away but rather to make it more widely available. "At a cost, of course, because the development doesn't happen for free," John says. But the introduction of the PVPA is a "good example of how the protection of intellectual property works for the benefit of farmers and consumers alike." Before PVPA was enacted, a company might introduce a new variety of soybean, and the next year other people could market the same variety without paying the company for its research efforts. Since PVPA, John says, "there has been a great increase in the money invested in soybean research and a faster rate of introduction of new and improved soybean varieties."

Do we need an ever-changing palette of new seed varieties? John says we do because "farming is almost always growing crops that aren't native to the place they're being planted. Corn is not native to the corn belt—prairie grasses are." So the crops that we grow for food, be they for animal feed or human consumption, are always in competition with native species. The plants man grows for his own purposes are vulnerable, then, to stresses that make them more vulnerable to disease, pest damage, and drought, or too much rain. "As the land continues to work, the pathogens and the insects continue to evolve themselves, to change, to overcome the defenses of the plants," says John.

Besides, he says, the virtues that the public wants in vegetables and other agricultural crops continue to change. We want carrots that are smoother and easier to clean, that are more tender, John says; man has always pushed to develop

new varieties to serve his own purposes, and corn and potatoes are two good examples of that.

A number of questions would have to be answered before this country could shift to a completely sustainable
method of producing food, John says. "It's been many
decades since we've seen a truly diverse and dispersed agriculture. One of the reasons that it's difficult to com-
pare bioengineered varieties with traditional varieties is that
we have adapted so many crops to be used in more specialized agriculture."

Who would work on these farms, if a "diverse and dispersed" system of agriculture were returned to the norm? "A
lot of people left agriculture because it's not an easy way to
make a living," John says. "It's dangerous to life and limb,
and it always has been. Many of those still farming are doing
so because they prefer an agricultural lifestyle—the benefits,
to them, outweigh the negative attributes." But most of us,
John believes, have rightly or wrongly decided that a farmer's
life is too hard. "If the trend were to reverse, I don't think
it's a safe assumption that people would necessarily flock to
the farm."

Consumers' buying habits, too, have changed the way
farming is done in this country, John says. How willing are
shoppers to return to an "unreliable and inconsistent, or nar-
rower, variety of availability?" he asks. The supply systems
have forced a new kind of relationship between the farmer
and the supplier, he says. Major retail grocers sign contracts
with produce distributors, who are obligated to provide a certain number of boxes of lettuce on a certain schedule, regard-
less of cost or supply. And growers are often forced to harvest
produce at a loss, to fulfill those contracts.

"What drives that, in the end, is the consumer demanding to have not only head lettuce, which may be of marginal
quality, but other lettuces, too, fifty-two weeks a year," says

John. "Will consumers change their desires? We certainly have a lot more choices than we used to, in terms of seasonal vegetables." But do consumers know how to use these vegetables, asks John rhetorically. In most cases, they seem not to know how.

In the end, says John, the similarities between the aims of bioengineering and the sustainable agriculture movement are greater than their differences. "I see almost universally a desire to do things in a way which is more sustainable," says John, "which uses the earth's resources more wisely, and which allows us to maintain a life we believe in and which we choose to live. I see a deep concern in the agricultural community about doing things in a way that's fundamentally better than the way we have to do things now. I think farmers are genuinely concerned about providing food that is nutritious and safe, and when available, farmers will choose options which allow them to achieve those goals."

As he tallies that list of goals, he doesn't see them as fundamentally different from those involved in the sustainable agriculture movement. "My job involves what other people call 'industrial agriculture,' but I can tell you that when I go out to the fields, I don't find people who are industries," John says. "I find people who are farmers. Certainly the market forces have caused consolidation. In many cases, people now farm land that is not their own. But in the end people are farming because they like that way of life and because they're concerned about doing that job well. The difference is not so much attitude as it is economic structure. It delivers a paycheck, and it provides a living."

The system is terribly complex, says John, but in the end, the goals of safe, nutritious food at affordable prices can be met with tools like bioengineering.

"Far from seeing biotechnology as being counter to the interests of sustainable agriculture, I see biotechnology as being critical to helping us move toward the ideal of sustain-ability," he says. "Since biotechnology is delivered through seeds, in our case, the technology inherently does not require large investments, specialized equipment, or capital invest-ments that are beyond the means of the farmer."

It's David Tricoli's job to develop the seeds that deliver Up-john's biotechnology. In 1992 David had a cumbersome title at Asgrow: tissue culture group leader in the experimental plant genetics division.

David spends his days in the quiet, serene surroundings of the lab at Asgrow's Kalamazoo headquarters. He works on the front lines of plant bioengineering, but his tools are recog-nizable to any high school science student: test tubes, scalpels, pipettes, petri dishes.

David is lean and slight; his movements convey compe-tence and confidence. He will show us how the mystery of plant bioengineering is done, as he tries—again—to create a strain of transgenic squash that reliably passes on its new traits to succeeding generations.

He takes up a squash seedling and removes the cotyle-dons—the first "leaves" of a seedling, which aren't true leaves, but which are especially rich in genetic material. He cuts the cotyledons into eight tiny pieces.

Plants created from cuttings of this sort are clones of the parent plant.

Next, David washes the pieces of cotyledon with a solu-tion rich in a kind of common bacteria found in soil. It's called *Agrobacterium tumefaciens*; *tumefaciens* means "tu-mor-causing," and in nature, the bacteria causes a plant dis-ease called crown gall. Nearly twenty-five years ago, scientists discovered that they could use *A. tumefaciens* as a sort of dump truck to carry new genetic material into plants. They did this by removing some of *A. tumefaciens*'s own genetic material and replacing it with whatever new material they wanted to insert in the plant under study. In David's case, *A. tumefaciens* carries coat proteins from several plant viruses that devastate squash plants. Inserting those proteins in the squash's genetic structure will make the squash immune to the diseases.

The squash cotyledons are cut up, David says, to provide "wound sites"—places where the bacteria can enter the plant's DNA. Then the cotyledon snippets are placed in an agar-filled Petri dish for a week or so to give *A. tumefaciens* time to do its work.

Next, the snippets are moved to another petri dish, the agar-enriched plant growth hormones. The goal is to encourage the cuttings to begin to grow into new plants. This isn't much different, David says, from pinning begonia leaves into the soil in hopes that they will root.

The growing medium is also laced with an antibacterial agent to kill the *A. tumefaciens*. It is no longer needed because it has done its job.

Again the little cuttings rest for about a week.

In that time some may begin to grow into new plants. Most, by far, won't; they'll end up in the bizarre-looking clumps that frustrated David when you first met him in the introduction. Those pieces of cotyledon didn't have the right genetic coding to program a new plant's growth.

Any successful pieces are transferred now to a third petri dish. The agar gel in this one is enhanced with an antibiotic that normally kills young plants. If the new plants survive, David knows that *A. tumefaciens* did its job. That's because he also inserted some genetic coding that gives plants resistance to this antibiotic; he sent that genetic material into the new little squash plants with the *A. tumefaciens* dump truck.

"It might take a thousand pieces before one takes

off," David says. "That's part of the frustration of this kind of science."

The long-shot survivors are coddled along in a high-tech plant nursery until they become full-fledged plants. At that stage they are treated the way you treat seedlings you've grown in preparation for your spring planting. They are gently acclimated to normal growing conditions, in the gardening process called "hardening off."

Research science is fascinating and frustrating, says David. "People talk about 'peak experiences.' There's the wonderment of discovering something new. You get to have those peak experiences quite often in this field. But along with that, you have to do a lot of mundane things, a lot of tedious things, every day. They say: 'Science is a dry orange. You have to squeeze it hard to get any juice.' The juice is there. You just have to work hard to get it."

Robyn Van En, whom we met previously when we talked about community-shared agriculture, is now living for the eleventh year on Indian Line Farm near Great Barrington, Massachusetts. Indian Line Farm is no longer a working CSA, Robyn says, because she spends most of her time as an organizer for CSA North America, of which she is the executive director. The community has taken to the community-shared agriculture concept, however. There are now some twenty CSAs within a twenty-mile radius of Indian Line Farm, the first CSA in the country.

Robyn is a native of Long Island and grew up in Southern California. After "a couple of years" of college, she says, she lived in South America and in other countries, and when she returned to the United States, she earned a living growing landscape perennials and vegetables.

She founded Indian Line Farm, she says, because when it came on the market, "I realized that it could be snatched up for development," a fate that has become commonplace in many other parts of Massachusetts, where land values skyrocketed during the early '80s. Old family farms were broken up for development in carefully planned subdivisions, where five or ten acres might be required for each house. That land is now lost permanently to agriculture, as Robyn points out.

The sixty-acre farm was called Indian Line because it's an old farm—the house is 150 years old, but the farm is far older than that—and it is just east of the New York state border. That border was, she says, literally "the Indian line": all the region's Native Americans lived in the West, which was to say in New York and beyond.

Robyn is familiar with all the arguments for bioengineering that John Sorenson puts forth. Perhaps because of her impassioned nature and machine-gun thinking, she does not agree with any of his theses.

"Farms have to be on a human scale," she says. "What we've got now is a bunch of 150-cow—or 500-cow—farms on what should be 50-cow farms. Each farm should develop itself to its highest potential, with its highest diversity. Most dairy farmers don't even have their own vegetable gardens anymore! Yet we were growing for three hundred people for forty-three weeks of the year on five acres of land; our members got fresh produce once a week all summer, and once a month, from the root cellar, all winter. And that was possible, even including a livable salary for the farmer and the part-timers."

The premise of sustainability is tied to regional growing, Robyn says. And right off the bat, regional growing decreases or eliminates the costs of trucking or flying foods long distances; it reduces fuel consumption for transportation; it eliminates the need for monocrop farms that use publicly subsidized water.

"Every state should look at its land," Robyn says. "They

should hold this land up as they look to the future of development. Agricultural land must be preserved. Concentrate on developing regional networks—or provincial networks, in Canada—and stop this trucking of food three thousand miles across the country, or even around the world. Forget the strawberries in November."

Regional growing improves the nutritional qualities of the foods we eat, Robyn says, because the food is fresher, eaten closer to where it was grown and sooner after it was harvested. A seasonal diet, composed of foods that are appropriate to the seasons in our climates, makes sure that we achieve balance and proper nutrition, she says. By eating a wider variety of foodstuffs we ensure ourselves against the maladies created by a limited diet.

Advances in solar technologies can make winter-season hothouses practical in colder climates for farmers who want to try that avenue, Robyn says. We will not automatically have to rely solely on dry beans and rutabagas in cold, long winters if we move to sustainable agriculture. But we do not have to truck foods long distances—nor use fragile fossil fuel resources—to feed ourselves.

And because long-distance transport is removed from the equation, Robyn elaborates, farmers can return to growing fruit and vegetable varieties that are selected for highest flavor, not longest shelf life. Plants bred for ease in mechanical harvesting lose their value, in comparison to other varieties, when mechanical harvesting isn't the goal. Many older varieties have been lost in a selection process that values long keeping above every other quality. Regional growing could return those varieties to household-name status. We could see a return to a country where different varieties are grown in different areas, which would enhance regional identities and contribute to the pleasures of traveling the country.

There is no shortage of food in the world, Robyn says.

There is plenty of food for everyone at the world's table. What's needed is better systems to see that the food we have gets to those who need it. "It's not countries growing millions of tons of grain to export or stockpile," she says. "It's local farms growing for local people."

According to Robyn, a sustainable farm gives back everything that's put into it. "There is a full nutrient base on the farm," she says, "along with components of companion planting—to host good bugs and birds—plus replenish the soil. So what's going on is that your soil is getting better, and your work is getting easier. In industrial agriculture we're using four hundred percent more pesticides than we did when they were first introduced—and only two percent of that gets to the bug. Yet we have not eliminated even one species of pest from our farms."

On sustainable farms there is no toxic overflow from the chemicals used to work the land, Robyn says. Issues of pesticide residues disappear completely when food is grown organically, eliminating a source of anxiety for parents who are concerned about their children's welfare. The land is safe from erosion because of integrated cropping practices; the visitor would see weed management and cleared ground, planted in crops that are suited to the terrain, the climate, and to each other.

Naturally, says Robyn, not every farm could produce every kind of foodstuff. Some farms are better suited to growing certain kinds of foods than others. But one way to address that is already happening. "One of the most exciting things about CSAs is coalitions of growers. One person is growing fruits and vegetables; someone else is milking cows; still another is raising chickens for meat and eggs. Each site is developed to its highest potential. If you have twenty acres of flat land, you don't grow twenty acres of vegetables. You put in an orchard, or you put in a vineyard, or you have some other things. The growers cooperate, rather than compete, because they know that their economic return is not based on selling their product for less than the guy next door. They know they can make a living, an honest, dignified living."

The landscape in Robyn's vision of a sustainable future looks very different from the one that John Sorenson sees. "You would see farm after farm," she says. "Life in those small rural communities would return, and they would be wonderful places to live again. The air would be clean all the time, not just on the days when they're not spraying. Birds would sing, and children could grow up knowing the names of the plants and animals in their regions because they would see them every day. Wildlife would return, in populations that the land could support, because watersheds would not be polluted, and farmers would leave some of their fields fallow each year in the name of improving the soil."

Moreover, says Robyn, all the people who lived nearby would have a better understanding of where their food comes from, how it is produced, and the kind of work that goes into its harvest. "I've seen adults whose eyes got as big as buttons when they see a carrot seedling or a lettuce seedling—they've never seen that in their lives," she says. "And it is transformative."

It will take time for us to make a transition to a completely sustainable form of agriculture, Robyn admits. But in the interim we could—we should—turn to community gardens and farmers' markets. "It's all regional production," she says. "It's keeping those dollars in the local economy, it's employing local people, it's keeping people on the land." And with the successes of local farmers markets, permanent buildings could be justified to make the markets even more accessible for more of the year. Market managers would handle marketing for the farmers, whose main work is growing food; managers would take care of public outreach so that the people in the community know when and where the market is open. Such markets, says Robyn, would be lively places, open several days each week and well attended whenever they are open. Farmers markets answer the people's need for choices. Community gardens bring them in touch with nature and with the weather and with each other.

Robyn concedes that food might be more expensive in a sustainable system, but its cost would reflect the real costs of production, not an artificially low cost that conceals worsening damage to the environment and to our health. She disagrees, however, with the idea that community-shared, sustainably-minded agriculture is "elitist" or "niche" marketing.

"It is accessible to everyone," she says firmly. "It doesn't matter whether you pay with cash or with food stamps or in work. This is all part of the flexibility of the community-shared agriculture idea. In Europe, people put away a dollar a day and plunk it down when the share payment is due. Just by having people share the farmer's risk, that big change affects how the farmer can do his job—and he can do it better in CSA. When he or she is paid once a year, the economic pressures are removed."

In tandem, sustainable agriculture practices and community-shared agriculture open farming opportunities to everyone—including people of color, women, and the developmentally, emotionally, or physically challenged, says Robyn. "It's a major breakthrough. It crosses all socioeconomic, ethnic, religious, and racial lines. It's win-win agriculture, for everybody involved."

Because the work is shared, no one is overburdened with the dangers and risks of agricultural living that John Sorenson mentions, she says. When economic fear is replaced by economic security, when toxic chemicals are not required for production, the farmer can concentrate on producing safe, nutritious food for everyone who counts on him or her to do so. And nonfarmers who help with the work learn to esteem that work, become familiar again with its intrinsic value.

John Sorenson sees a future in which farmers, whether owners or employees, are still businessmen. His future accommodates the needs of business and incorporates those needs in food production for the people of this country.

Robyn Van En sees a future where the emphasis is on cooperation between people, where the land is honored and nurtured, and the food produced is shared equally among all who need it.

They are very different visions, two in the millions of possible futures from which we might choose. Whose vision is closer to the future that you want to see?

# 9

# *Voting with Your Buck*

*Y*ou've seen in the preceding chapters how the values of the men and women who grow your food differ. You've seen, also, two very different views of what the future might hold for us, depending on how we decide to raise the food we need for ourselves and other countries. Now it's time to talk about how your grocery money can make a difference and how you can shape our future.

Your decisions will be easiest if you support the aims of industrial agriculture, with its increasing reliance on bioengineering. Buy new products as they come to market; write letters to your local newspapers, to the FDA, to local, state, and federal government agencies monitoring or regulating bioengineered foods. Your support is crucial to the companies that believe these products have promise for the new era we enter.

Tell the supermarket manager and the chef in your favorite restaurant why you feel the way you do, and don't hesitate to be vocal: they want and need to know how you feel about this topic.

Those of you who choose to support a more strictly sustainable vision have different challenges. We'll explore the ways in which you can cast your vote in the coming pages, and we'll discuss why your habits may need to change if you feel strongly about the way your food is grown.

We will talk about food in two arenas: at home and away from home—in restaurants, take-out places, and the like.

## FOOD AT HOME

The hardest change for many of us is to begin—or learn—to cook again. We find it easiest to rely on others to prepare our food because we say we haven't the time to cook ourselves. In turning over this responsibility for our own welfare to strangers, we endorse a system that transports foodstuffs thousands of miles, subjects that food to myriad manipulations, and charges us for the privilege of doing so, even while few of the profits reach the farmer.

Many of us feel that we can't possibly find time to cook fresh ingredients from scratch. I would argue that this isn't so: most of the cuisines of the world include dishes that don't take much prep or cooking time. The stir-fries of China are a good example: because fuel is costly in China, these are dishes that take only moments to cook. Pasta, soups, tortilla-based dishes—none take long to prepare.

When people tell me that they don't have time to cook, I wonder what they *do* have time for. The answer can be found in many rooms of most of our homes: television. Tired at the end of hectic days, we can only sag onto a couch or into an easy chair. It's no coincidence that ice cream and dessert commercials predominate in prime-time programming. Those ads are timed to appear just about the time we begin to want a bedtime snack.

What people mean when they say they don't have time to cook is that they don't think cooking is important or pleasurable enough to warrant an investment of their energy and time.

Yet in cultures where food is highly prized, its preparation takes on the form of family ritual. Many hands join in mealtime proceedings, and the food that the family prepares is accorded dignity and respect because every member knows the work that went into the meal. In most cultures food is seen as precious; eating together is the measure of friendship for many of the world's peoples.

Families with small children often find especially difficult challenges when it's time to cook dinner. I think that is partly because we no longer require children to join in the preparation of their own meals. Toddlers can place potato peelings in the compost bucket without danger of harm; older children can wash and peel and cut up vegetables. Teens can be taught to prepare meals or assemble casseroles for freezing, to join in planning the family's menus, and help with the shopping. In the process, children who learn about cooking learn, too, that their family values food and considers its treatment important. They grow up knowing how to feed themselves well, into the bargain.

Enticing your children into the kitchen is easy. Cooking is essentially a sensual act, and its fascinating aromas, textures, and tastes intrigue children. For a youngster there is an aspect of magic in cooking: how do flour, shortening, sugar, eggs, and milk turn into a cake? The arts of food preparation are accessible to everyone of every level of capability. But someone has to teach children how to prepare food. I think it should be their parents.

In teaching a cooking class to a group of Girl Scouts ages eleven to thirteen, I found to my amazement that not five of the sixty girls knew how to peel a potato. They didn't know how to hold the peeler, and they didn't know how to hold the potato. They didn't know how to inspect the potato and cut away bruised or spoiled spots. Yet virtually all said they helped their parents prepare their suppers. How could that be?

Further questions revealed that they believed microwaving a frozen dinner was cooking. Indeed, many of those Scouts didn't know that potatoes can be baked, roasted, steamed, boiled, fried, or broiled. No one had shown those curious young women how versatile a raw potato can be and how different it tastes depending on how it is cooked.

*Cooking for yourself and your family is the first key act in a life that supports farmers struggling to stay on the land.* When you prepare a meal with your own hands, you add the "value" that you previously paid a manufacturer to add for you. Less of the price of your food goes to middlemen like distributors, brokers, manufacturers, and processors; more of its price is returned to the farmer who grew it. This is especially true if the food has been grown or raised locally so that packers and shippers have not added their costs.

Cooking from scratch is more economical than buying manufactured foods. It also allows you to add other values to your meals: the value of honest work, both yours and the grower's; the values of emotional, physical, and spiritual nurturing.

Cooking from whole ingredients has unexpected boons for your health: most of the fat, cholesterol, and sodium we eat are found in heavily processed, fast-food products, and much of it is hidden from us in foods like cookies and canned soups and sandwiches, because we didn't prepare the foods ourselves. Cooking whole foods returns your control over your body's nutritional needs; it restores to you the power to manage your fat, cholesterol, and sodium consumption.

Virtually every community offers cooking classes in community-education programs; cookware and department stores, too, often offer classes. Learning new skills or honing your existing ones will help you feed your family faster at the end of a busy day—without relying on packaged, value-added foods.

To cook well and quickly at home, you need wholesome, good-quality ingredients, as close as possible to their natural state. An easy way to find them is to buy as many of your groceries as you can from the perimeter of the store. The aisles up and down are stocked with manufactured and prepared products, and it is those products that may account for most of your grocery dollar.

But you still need to think about what you buy and whether it accurately reflects your values.

Many of us have turned to selecting organic produce out of disgust with and fear of the potential dangers posed by our chemical-dependent agricultural system. It is true that organic farming is an important step toward sustainability, but it is also true that most of the organic produce sold in the city of New York is shipped in from California. The produce is transported across the country using the same energy-gobbling systems that its industrial counterpart has adopted. The key to sustainability is many small producers on land throughout the country. But local growers can't make a go of it financially if they are compelled to compete with big concerns, even organic ones, whose size permits them to manipulate market prices in their favor.

So try to buy, whenever possible, locally grown organically produced produce and meats. Don't be surprised if you find this difficult. The manager of my favorite grocery store told me he would love to stock and sell Michigan-grown produce but couldn't do so for two reasons. The first is that his customers will not surrender their desire for out-of-season produce. As a result the produce brokers who sell to him have him over a barrel: they know he needs lettuce and tomatoes in winter, so they threaten not to sell to him in winter if he doesn't stock their produce in summer. I think of that each August when I see Florida sweet corn and California plums on his produce counters, instead of Michigan fruits and vegetables.

The other reason he can't stock locally grown produce is because he thinks there are no longer enough Michigan farmers growing vegetables and fruit and producing milk and meat to fill his demand, even in season. He has had the very devil of a time, he says, trying to locate sources for locally grown, organic produce and getting that produce into his store in appealing condition. And even when he has been able to offer local fruits and vegetables, shoppers often pass them over in favor of produce that looks picture perfect. His customers forget, perhaps, that foods grown without chemicals may not be as photogenic as industrial-style produce. They forget that "a blemish can be a promise," as sustainable agriculture advocate Laura DeLind says.

The curious thing is that many Michigan growers raise exactly the kind of produce he says he wants to buy. But my grocer hasn't seen the value in locating these sources and solving problems that might accompany getting their produce from farm to market. His customers haven't told him that they want locally grown, organic produce. He is a shrewd businessman in a very competitive business; I believe that his customers' silence has given him a false impression, but I also believe that he would respond in an instant if he began to detect a demand from his customers for locally grown produce.

So there are two things to remember in this part of your grocery store visit.

If you don't see locally grown organic foodstuffs, ask to speak to the store manager and tell him that's what you want. He may answer you with a number of reasons why fulfilling your request isn't possible or even reasonable; don't be dismayed or dissuaded. Remember: you've got what he wants—your money.

Also, strive to eat fresh seasonal vegetables and locally grown foodstuffs whenever possible. Remember that your choice to buy pallid winter tomatoes is part of the reason why your home state's fresh produce isn't in your stores, and your choice of a frozen vegetable in a synthetic "butter" sauce lessens the share of your grocery dollar that goes to the farmer who grew the vegetable in the first place. Dozens of interesting vegetables are in season even in the dead of winter in the northern states: kale, fennel, parsnips, and the families of winter squashes. You won't go hungry, and your family will benefit from both the nutritional variety and the broadened knowledge of the many kinds of vegetables available.

Of course, it is unlikely that your state grows every food you need. Coffee is not grown in Georgia; Minnesota is not known for its olive trees and oils. But perhaps you will find, as I have, that you are more sparing with those items when you have thought about where they came from and who profits from your purchase.

If your supermarket manager is not responsive to your requests for more locally grown foods, you may wonder where you'll find the foods you need.

Shop at farmers markets whenever possible. Here the link between the people who grow your food and your grocery dollar is the closest: in many cases, you're buying directly from the grower herself. Most medium-to-large cities and many smaller ones have year-round farmers markets. If you don't know where your nearest farmers market is, call your state's Department of Agriculture or your county extension service office, which is a public service arm of your state's agricultural college. Many growers who sell their foodstuffs at farmers markets already use or are moving in the direction of sustainable agricultural practices; these struggling farmers need your support if you value their labor and their nurturing attitudes toward the land. Note that some farmers markets permit vendors to sell produce that they themselves have not grown but have instead bought at wholesale houses. Common sense will tell you that a vendor in a Wisconsin farmers market is unlikely to have raised the grapefruit you see in January. Does that reflect your values of seasonality, wholesomeness, and local production?

Join or form a community-supported agriculture farm. As you saw with Bruce Schultz, Will Raap, and Robyn Van En, CSAs are a vibrant, exciting way for you to help a grower stay on the land—and feed yourself well in the process. Most CSA growers are already sustainably minded and follow organic farming practices and humane livestock treatment. CSAs can help your children learn about the beginnings of their food; by working in the CSA gardens just a few times each season, they will come to understand the work that goes into growing food. Your children will be less likely to waste food if they know firsthand how much effort it took to raise it. And they may more eagerly adopt new foods if they see them growing.

The CSA movement is still fledgling in this country. Your state's Department of Agriculture and/or your county's cooperative extension service offices are two places to begin in your search to locate an existing CSA. Or you can contact CSA North America, listed in the resources for this book. While you're speaking to those agencies, ask if there is an organic farming association in your state. If no CSAs are in operation in your area, ask for help in locating a farmer who might be willing to establish one. Check, too, with the agricultural department at your state's land-grant universities; many state agriculture colleges have begun to fund research in sustainable methods (although most of their research money is directed to conventional agricultural practices). Information on how to establish a CSA is available from the sources listed, too.

It may be a frustrating, complex struggle that proceeds in fits and starts; one woman told me that she invested five years in seeing a CSA in her area begun, but it is now running smoothly. Or it may go as easily as the organization of the Indian Line CSA in Massachusetts.

Take part in community garden programs in your area, and if none are available, help start one. Many cities have begun programs that allow citizens to lease a garden space for a small fee. These community gardens, sometimes tucked away in low-income neighborhoods and sometimes in city parks or vacant lots, foster a sense of neighborliness among the gardeners, and they grow much more than food: they grow friendships. It's hard to resist striking up a conversation with the gardener next to you when his tomatoes look so much better than your own. Coming together in the common goal of growing fruits and vegetables promotes a sense of belonging and community. Experienced gardeners welcome the chance to teach newcomers, and there is a rich lode of knowledge to be tapped in our community members who have gardened, often organically, for many years.

Surplus foods from community gardens are often donated to community feeding programs, so foods grown there never need go to waste.

A community garden program begins with convincing your community's government that there is a need for and an interest in such a project. It requires little money to start since the land is publicly owned, the community often has the heavy equipment to prepare the gardens in the first year, and the low fees charged for each plot will generally cover the costs of the labor involved. Seeds and seedlings may sometimes be obtained as donations, but are inexpensive even if they must be purchased. The most difficulty may seem to be in locating a group of people who will agree to participate. Talk to your friends and neighbors. Propose the idea to the congregation of your church. Enlist the students in your schools.

While this option does little for struggling farmers, it does provide you and your family with wholesome foods produced in sustainable ways, and it does much to reduce your support for industrial agricultural food systems.

Consult the resource list in the back of this book for sources of seeds that are not hybridized and that preserve agricultural diversity. As more and more plant varieties are patented by agrochemical and agribusiness companies, these "heirloom" varieties become more and more valuable. Learning how to save seeds from year to year is not difficult, but you can't save the seeds from hybrid plants: there is no certainty that the next generation will grow into the plant you expect.

Find and patronize U-pick and farmstand operations whenever possible. These operations usually advertise in the classified sections of daily and weekly newspapers; you may be surprised to find how many such places are within an hour's drive of your home, even if you live in a major city. Talk to the growers to find out whether their products are raised using sustainable approaches. In some cases you may find a grower who wants to learn more about organic and sustainable methods; your support and encouragement may mean the difference between his success and his failure. If he or she is reluctant or unwilling to consider those methods, explain why you think the change is important.

You may be interested in canning, freezing, or drying some of the fresh produce you get from your CSA or community garden or buy from farmstands and U-pick farms. If you don't know how to do this, or if you haven't done so in many years, please consult a recently published book, or contact your county extension service's home economist for advice. Preserving food for long storage takes special care in preparation and practice; although it is not difficult to do, it can be dangerous if not done properly. Old practices have changed in many cases, and it is prudent to be sure that your method is deemed safe. Food preservation is a lot of work, albeit worthwhile; it would be silly to spend all that time and effort only to have to discard your rewards.

Finally, decrease your reliance on manufactured and prepared foods. Remember that the farmer's share of your grocery dollar is directly diminished by every set of hands your food passes through. Study your buying habits. Fresh locally grown broccoli in a cheese sauce made with milk, a flour-and-butter roux, and some grated Cheddar tastes far better than fresh broccoli drenched in "pasteurized processed cheese food" heated in the microwave and poured over the vegetable. It is superior, too, to frozen broccoli packaged with a heat-and-eat cheese sauce made from milk proteins and whey by-products, with lots of preservatives and sodium. And your children will learn what broccoli can and should taste like, rather than having their palates conditioned to the manipulated flavors of processed foods.

Use manufacturers' coupons sparingly and wisely. While couponing is a good way to trim your grocery bills, remember that coupons are produced by food processors whose motivation is to convince you to spend extra money on their products. They're betting that once you've tried their "new-

and-improved" product, you'll pick it up the next time and the next from habit—even without the coupons. Couponing, then, can give you a false sense of economy: you're paying less money for foods that may have been overpriced to begin with.

If you are an avid couponer, the next time you go to the grocery store, notice which edible items on your shopping list *don't* have cents-off coupons to go with them; it's a safe bet that they're foodstuffs that are whole, unprocessed, and unmanipulated.

Remember, too, that national-label meat products like already-sliced turkey cutlets and boneless skinless chicken breasts arrive at your market through a system that you may not support. You may find your own values closer to those of a local poultry producer who counts on you to know the basic kitchen skills necessary to bone a breast or slice a cutlet.

## FOOD AWAY FROM HOME

We eat a lot of our meals away from home, and we start early: many children take both breakfast *and* lunch at school. It's easier, we say, to buy lunch than it is to pack and carry one; we may not be satisfied with what we eat, but at least it didn't cost us much effort. Yet the only bargain in fast foods is that they're fast. Their quality is in no way equal to that of the foods you prepare at home; they are higher in unhealthful nutrients like fat, cholesterol, and sodium than we need, and they are lower in nutrients like fiber, vitamins, and minerals than we would wish.

The companies that sell hamburgers and tacos may not be companies whose policies we endorse and support. Remember that much of the beef used in fast-food sandwiches is raised in Central America, and remember, too, that McDonald's is the world's largest buyer of beef from slaughtered dairy cows that may have been injected with rBST/rBGH. The single leaf of iceberg lettuce on your fast-food hamburger came from a monocrop farm, probably in California or Arizona or Florida; it was raised using hundreds of pounds of chemical fertilizers, pesticides, and herbicides, and it drank gallons of irreplaceable water before it ever left the farm. Getting it from those farms to your nearest restaurant used thousands of gallons of gasoline to fuel truck, jet, and railroad engines. After it was prepared by strangers' hands, that food was packaged in energy-gobbling plastic and over-wraps of cardboard and paper; while much of it is recyclable, most of it ends up on your streets or in your local landfill. And most of the profit from your purchase went not to the farmer but to the franchise's owner.

Your children may not understand why your values don't encourage fast-food meals and prepackaged treats. Talk to older children and explain why you've reached your decisions; sweeten younger children's dismay by teaching them to pack lunches that include their own wholesome favorites.

It may be a struggle, especially at first. But you teach best by your own example, and empower your children with the courage and strength to resist peer pressure.

A mother of several children told me that she caved in to her children's demand that she stop packing her homemade applesauce in their lunches. Their friends, she said, carried plastic-wrapped prepackaged applesauce and puddings, and the friends teased her children. The mother made her decision based on her concern about her children's happiness; but in doing so, she may have taught them that their friends' values and opinions were more important than her own. Perhaps she might have instead explained to them the reasons why she could not support their request for commercially prepared snacks; she might have helped her children develop responses to the teasing, so they would feel stronger in defending their own family's values.

Eat in restaurants whose chefs and cooks are members of the Pure Food Campaign's boycott of genetically engineered foods or are members of the national coalition called Chefs: 2000. Some two thousand chefs across the country have already declared their support for sustainability by joining one or both of these organizations; they need to know that you support their decision. These chefs, some powerful and nationally known, others with more local reputations, have vowed that they will not serve bioengineered foods and that they will strive to serve only locally grown, seasonable ingredients. Let them know that you appreciate their work. You'll find the addresses of both the Pure Food Campaign and of Oldways Preservation & Exchange Trust, which sponsors Chefs: 2000, in the resources list at the back of this book.

Don't order foods out of season, and decline to eat them if they are served to you. Raspberries have come to be a signature garnish on desserts served at upscale restaurants. Yet most of the fresh raspberries sold during the winter are imported from Chile, where they are grown on land that has been converted from the production of food for local people. The chef in your favorite restaurant will continue to pay the exorbitant prices for these fragile out-of-season fruits if he thinks his customers want them. But he'll stop very quickly when he sees plate after plate returned to the kitchen with the expensive raspberries untouched. The same is true, naturally, for out-of-season lettuces in salads and vegetables flown in from other states. Restaurant owners are alert to what their customers want.

Be patient with restaurants struggling to change their supply systems. Since so much of this country's "infrastructure"—the delivery routes, the supply lines, and the packaging or processing plants for meat and dairy goods—has been lost, it sometimes may be frustrating for both you and the restaurateur as she tries to locate sustainable sources for foodstuffs. You can help her by understanding if the special you wanted isn't available or if there are no tomatoes on the salad.

Share knowledge with your favorite restaurant's staff. If you've located a wonderful source for top-quality foodstuffs nearby, tell your favorite chef. She may be able to work with the grower to supply the restaurant. And the grower whose products you like would probably love to hear about a nearby chef who may be interested in his crop.

Eat in locally owned restaurants, and try to eat regional foods when you travel. It used to be true that many of the resorts in Hawaii featured restaurants that served "continental" cuisine, prepared from ingredients flown thousands of miles to be used in kitchens by people who didn't value the good ingredients they had growing outside their back doors. Now a legion of young, creative, energetic Hawaiian chefs has come to prize the myriad riches of the islands' own supplies; the result is a dynamic, healthful, satisfying style of cooking that is as bright and charming as the islands themselves. If you travel there, you're likely to find taro in many forms. Eating and appreciating the foods of another culture is among the fastest ways to understand how that culture sees the world.

The rise of national and international food manufacturing companies has directly contributed to the loss of rich regionality in America's cookery, both public and private. And the press to ensure absolute consistency in ingredients' taste—as in McDonald's push to compel its European franchises to use tomatoes grown from American seed, rather than from native varieties—has worsened the danger of decreasing biodiversity. McDonald's goal is to have every single hamburger served anywhere in the world taste exactly like every other hamburger it serves; that may not be a value you hold dear.

These are just a few ways you can express your values with your food dollars; I'm certain that you'll discover more. Hundreds of millions of dollars are spent each year to convince you to believe in the value of manufactured, processed foods. The secret to resisting this heavy pressure is to think of who will profit by your buying decisions. You may have come to believe that the person whose labor and love for the land produced the food you eat should be the person who profits most.

Farmers don't advertise much.

They're too busy working.

# Resources

Here are some resources to begin to reconnect with farmers and the people who produce the foods you eat. Check with your state's Department of Agriculture, headquartered in your state's capital, for contacts and addresses for organic growers' associations and other sustainable agriculture organizations near you.

## COMMUNITY-SUPPORTED AGRICULTURE AND COMMUNITY GARDENS

American Community Gardening Association
325 Walnut Street
Philadelphia, PA 19106
(215) 625-8280

> Information about community gardens that belong to the association nationwide.

Biodynamic Farming Association
Box 550
Kimberton, PA 19442

> Publishes a list of CSAs and training opportunities across the country.

Committee for Sustainable Agriculture
P.O. Box 1300
Colfax, CA 95713
(916) 346-2777

> Sponsors the annual Ecological Farming Conference, publishes *Organic Food Matters* newspaper, offers educational and networking support.

CSA North America
Indian Line Farm
RR3, Box 85, Jug End Road
Great Barrington, MA 01230

> Send $10 for a list of resources for starting and running a CSA, plus a directory of existing CSAs (includes postage and handling).

Healthy Harvest Society
1424 16th Street NW, Suite 105
Washington, DC 20036
(202) 462-8800

> Publishes a bimonthly newsletter and the *Directory of Sustainable Agriculture*. Develops programs for information and research, developing organic markets, food and nutrition policy.

International Alliance for Sustainable Agriculture
Newman Center, University of Minnesota
1701 University Avenue SE
Minneapolis, MN 55414
(612) 331-1099

> Nonprofit, tax-exempt organization founded by farmers, consumers, researchers, business leaders, government officials, and others. Publishes a quarterly newsletter, *Manna*, and many books and other publications.

Rodale Institute
33 East Minor Street
Emmaus, PA 18098
(215) 683-6383

> Publishes *Organic Gardening* magazine; conducts research through experimental gardens at the institute

### BOOKS ABOUT GROWING AND PREPARING FOOD

*Cooking from a Garden* by Rosalind Creasy, Sierra Club Books, 1988.

> Features recipes for seasonal and ancient foodstuffs.

*From the Good Earth: A Celebration of Growing Food Around the World* by Michael Abelman, Abrams, 1993.

*Green Groceries* by Jeanne Heifetz, HarperCollins, 1992.

> Mail-order sources for organic foods.

*Rainforest in Your Kitchen* by Martin Teitel, Island Press, 1992.

Practical tips on creating environmental change through the foods you eat.

*Recipes from an Ecological Kitchen* by Lorna J. Sass, Morrow, 1992.

No-meat recipes that emphasize unprocessed, unmanipulated foods.

## BOOKS ABOUT AGRICULTURE AND ALTERNATIVE SYSTEMS

*Alternative Agriculture* by the National Research Council, 1988.

Fairly technical, this review of NRC's Board on Agriculture findings examines in close detail 14 farms where alternative practices are working well.

*Farms of Tomorrow: Community Supported Farms, Farm Supported Communities* by Trauger M. Groh and Steven S. H. McFadden.

Available by mail from the Bio-dynamic Farming Association, address above.

*From Land to Mouth* by Brewster Kneen, NC Press, updated edition, 1993.

Available by mail ($25 American covers shipping and handling) from The Ram's Horn, 125 Highfield Road, Toronto, Ontario M41 2T9 Canada. Subscriptions to *The Ram's Horn*, published 11 times yearly, are $20.

*Healthy Harvest—A Global Directory of Sustainable Agriculture and Horticultural Organizations*, Potomac Valley Press, 1993.

*Seeds of Change: The Living Treasure* by Kenny Ausubel, HarperSan Francisco, 1994.

> An impassioned argument on the importance of biodiversity, along with an explanation of why seed-saving for traditional plants is important.

## ORGANIZATIONS FOR CHEFS AND OTHERS

Chefs: 2000
Oldways Preservation and Exchange Trust
45 Milk Street
Boston, MA 02109
(617) 695-0600

> A national coalition of chefs dedicated to sustainability and the right to safe, wholesome food for all people. Oldways Preservation and Exchange Trust has been described as a "food issues think tank"; it is dedicated to the principles of biodiversity and sustainability.

The Pure Food Campaign
1130 17th Street NW, Suite 630
Washington, DC 20036
(202) 775–1132

> Organized by Jeremy Rifkin's Foundation on Economic Trends, the Pure Food Campaign boycotts bioengineered foods as unnecessary and potentially dangerous to the environment, the consumer, and the planet.

# Index

growth methods, 54
joining or forming a CSA farm, 182–84
lower income shareholders, 59
newsletters, 59–60
the origins of, 62–64
output of, 56–57
premise of, 52
problems encountered by, 58–60
resources, 191–93
sharer's role, 53–54
site use, 171
spiritual aspect of, 57–58, 65–66
work load, distribution of, 54
Composting, 8, 68, 69, 128, 177
Consumers, 9–10
attitudes toward bioengineered foods, 4, 15, 92
buying habits of, 164–65
industrial agriculture, ways of supporting, 175–76
knowing where food comes from, 1–2, 172
seasonal diet, eating a, 170, 180, 181
sustainable agriculture, ways of supporting, *see* Sustainable agriculture, ways of supporting
*Cooking from a Garden* (Creasy), 193
Cooking whole foods at home, 176–79
classes on, 179
as family effort, 177–78
health benefits of, 178–79
Cooperatives, dairy, 101–03
Cornell University, 111
*Corporate Reapers: The Book of Agribusiness, The* (Krebs), 10
County extension service, 182, 185
Coupons, manufacturers', 185–86

Cows:
bioengineered hormone to increase milk production of, 12, 74, 80, 84–94, 108–11, 187
*see also* Dairying; Livestock
Creasy, Rosalind, 193
Crichton, Michael, 18
Crittendon, Dr. Lyman, 121
Crop insurance, 22
Crop rotation, 82
Crown gall, 166
CSA North America, 168, 182
address of, 191

Dairying, 73–113
bioengineered hormone injected in cows to increase milk production, 12, 74, 80, 84–93, 108–11, 187
breeding by artificial insemination, 79
cooperatives, dairy, 101–03
family dairy farmer, 95–97, 103–08, 110–13
federal price support programs, 98–100
feeding of cows, 81–82, 91, 107
herd management, 77–78, 91
marketing of milk, 97–103
milking, 112
milk production per cow, 97–98
pricing of milk, underpinnings of, 97–103
processors, 100–01, 103
segregating cows by age, 78
sustainable approach to, 95–97, 103–08, 111–13
DeLind, Laura, 180
*Detroit News, The*, 18
Dickinson, Mike, 91
Disease resistance, transgenic crops with increased, 160, 161, 162, 167

### · A NOTE ON THE TYPE ·

The typeface used in this book is a version of Bodoni, based on the fonts cut by the Italian printer Giambattista Bodoni (1740–1813) at the turn of the nineteenth century. Early in his career his work was conventional (though he was always forward-looking and was an admirer of the work of John Baskerville), but as a product of his time, Bodoni believed that type design ought to be rational. Late in life he produced the revolutionary fonts named for him, the first of the so-called "moderns," characterized by high contrast between thin and thick strokes and "unbracketed" (untapered), thin, right-angled serifs. For the first time, type left behind both the chisel and the quill, so *modern* is an appropriate term: Once typography was free of its roots in engraving and calligraphy (and despite the disapproval of the likes of William Morris), an explosion of variation in letter forms started, one that has continued ever since.